FIT FOR A KING

Fit for a King

SUE BARNETT

KINGSWAY PUBLICATIONS
EASTBOURNE

ISBN 0 86065 322 6

Unless otherwise indicated, biblical quotations are from
the New International Version, © New York International
Bible Society 1978.

GNB = Good News Bible
      © American Bible Society 1976

AV = Authorized Version
      Crown copyright

Front cover photo: Art Directors Photolibrary—London

Chapter 4 is based on material by the author
which originally appeared in Marion Stroud
(ed.), *Prayer is a Way of Life* (Marshalls 1984).

Printed in Great Britain for
KINGSWAY PUBLICATIONS LTD
Lottbridge Drove, Eastbourne, E.Sussex BN23 6NT by
Richard Clay (The Chaucer Press) Ltd, Bungay, Suffolk.
Typeset by Nuprint Services Ltd, Harpenden, Herts.

IN MEMORY OF
JOY
AND WITH GRATITUDE
TO
BOB, JOHN, ROB & ANDY

CONTENTS

ACKNOWLEDGEMENTS

Thank you to Wendy Normandale for typing the manuscript and for her patience and skill in interpreting the scribbled draft.

To John and Ruth Arkell for their prayerful support, understanding friendship and continuous encouragement to keep going when I felt like giving up.

To my parents, without whom this book could never have been written.

And most of all to Doug, Stephen and Duncan for their inspiration, patience and love.

1

FIT FOR LIFE

I have always found a tracksuit the most comfortable form of clothing. That third night curled up by Joy's bed was no exception. The lights had been dimmed, voices were lowered. The silence was punctuated by the irregular breathing of a very brave lady holding onto life by a faint gasp, determined to see her fifty-fourth birthday.

Although my eyes were on her fading form, my mind raked through the previous months of precious memories when Joy's eyes had been open and twinkling, cheeky and cross. The fun she had made of my massaging her stiffening legs, and tonging her wayward hair, fully realizing that her physical life was slipping away fast.

Another desperate intake of breath brought me back to the tiny hospital room, our home for the past long days and nights. Her youngest son Andrew, whose sixteen years hung heavy that night, eased his aching arm as he tightened his hold on his Mum's hand. The contrast between his strong, tanned fingers, normally grasping life with all its opportunity and promise, and the chill hand lying now in his clasp, cut painfully across my memories, and my gaze crept slowly back to her face, lit by a pool of dimmed light.

Her illness had brought her a lot of pain and weakness, but it had also been a time when she had experienced the tireless love and comfort of her family of men who had nursed her right to the end.

As Joy waited patiently for the long days to crawl by, she discovered a new friend, who had also endured a long and painful death, who understood the empty hours of despair, frustration and loneliness and who had the answers to all the questions throbbing through her aching mind. As drugs dimmed Joy's twinkling eyes, her confidence was in a God willing to clothe himself in a human body, who had committed himself to a premature death at the age of thirty-three, thus enabling her to have life beyond those closing months. Life without pain, tears, despair and death.

Joy clung onto the words we found in 2 Corinthians chapter four verse sixteen in the Good News Bible:

. . . we never become discouraged. Even though our physical being is gradually decaying, yet our spiritual being is renewed day after day.

A new spiritual life had been born within Joy's dying physical body and it was this fresh, new Joy who peacefully left her earthly cloak just two short minutes before her birthday was over.

How thankful I was that she had discovered what eternal life was all about. As I left the hospital in the chill early hours, and found the world sleeping on, peacefully, oblivious of the quiet exit Joy had made, a sadness swept through me. Not for Joy, but for the thousands soon to be waking to the breakfast shows, physical fitness, and stars predictions, to diet-conscious breakfasts, and exercise routines. We live in a world so aware of the physical body—we exercise it, we feed it, we pamper it, we clothe it, we sauna it, we paint it, we measure it, we weigh it, we massage it, we sun it, we exploit it, we sell it, and then eventually—we leave it!

God intended us to enjoy our lives. He sent his Son Jesus who said:

> I have come that they may have life, and have it to the full (Jn 10:10).

But if we persistently care for our physical being and neglect our spiritual being, we miss out on what real life is all about.

Looking back over years of sport and competitions, P.E. College and keep-fit classes, I loved every minute of the discipline and team spirit, and these had influenced and enriched my life as a teacher, wife and Mum, as a friend and neighbour. Above all I realized that God had taken the very ability that he gave me physically to deepen and invigorate my spiritual life. I shared some of these thoughts with Joy over endless cups of coffee. I share them now with you and her family. It may be over a cup of coffee, on the top of a bus, in your living room, on the beach. Whenever and wherever you read this book, be quiet for a moment and think over the life and care of your body, both physically and spiritually.

2

FIT FOR BATTLE

At the height of the summer of 1942 a commanding officer sat bathing his aching feet after a route march with his men in Durham. One of them now stood to attention in front of him. 'Compassionate leave? What for, Raymond?' Without hesitation, Corporal Raymond replied, 'I have just been informed I have another daughter, sir.' After a moment's consideration, leave was granted and my father was travelling impatiently down to London where my mother was struggling with her disappointment. Having been informed before the birth that she was to have twins, her heart was set on boys to complete her family of girls. Her weakness was so acute it was the doctor who suggested the name Susan and I have been plain Sue, with no middle name, ever since.

I was born into a loving family, who quickly adapted to three girls, later four, and into a wartorn Britain and battle-scarred London. When the great exodus from the cities occurred, my mother set up home in the cellar under our house. The coal was piled dustily one end, a camp bed and cot the other. Provisions, in case we were buried, were always at hand but we escaped injury, although five adjoining houses were flattened. The

Battle of Britain and the Blitz forged amongst the British people, and especially Londoners, such a unity that seemed sufficient to withstand anything future years might hold. These were the years of my earliest recollections.

Soon after my birth, my father was posted to Egypt. He returned to a three-year-old daughter who had idolized his uniformed photographs and my mother's graphic descriptions. However, there is a world of difference between pictures and a real, live person. I sat staring suspiciously at this strange man. I am told the extent of my welcome was whispered in my mother's ear, 'He hasn't got much hair, has he?' The end of the war and the years immediately following coloured my life considerably. The relief of survival after years of turmoil, and living in a Britain free of war, was a precious inheritance shared with me by a thankful family. The winds of war had swept through our country, but they had only just started raging in my heart and life as I grew up. The battle was very much on!

Just eighteen short months after victory was declared in Europe, I was marched, not so victoriously, into my first classroom. My kaleidoscope of memories includes battles with sewing which bore no resemblance to hemming, the comforting, fur-coated playground lady, fidgeting angels in the nativity play, and kiss chase around the annex buildings! My primary school was at the foot of a hill over which Wandsworth prison towered. The hollow chime of the bell, announcing another hanging, followed by the heavy silence that hung over the area, echoes in my memory. These moments of stillness were very few, as I literally tumbled through life, bouncing from one obstacle to the next, scaling problems like the trees on my favourite playground, Wandsworth Common. I took the knocks and gave my fair share. My parents had given me life and at the time I didn't debate or question it—I just got on and lived it.

Living meant eating and our house was a haven of delicious home cooking. To this day the smells wafting from the kitchen hold the strongest memories. Garden mint boiling with new potatoes, freshly baked cakes, hot from the oven, bread toasted by the coal fire, and summer fruit from the garden gently bubbling on the stove.

'Dig for Britain' we were urged and every spare piece of ground sprouted vegetables and every window sill ripened tomatoes. Late fruit, obstinately staying green, found its way into delicious chutney which, carefully guarded, could last until enjoyed with cold turkey on Boxing Day. Christmas always triggers off a mixture of memories. Security, warmth, excitement and expectation. Yet along with the chutney on Boxing Day crept a niggling disappointment that the heady excitement so rapidly evaporated into pine-needled carpets and limp decorations, torn wrapping paper and broken toys.

Long anticipated birthdays came and went and the pleasant pattern of my early years became interwoven with disjointed strands of uneasiness. The security of being a lively part of a family and its activities was replaced by an isolated unrest. I began to flex my strengthening muscles of individuality and the battle of independence catapulted me into my teens. Struggles with parents, sisters, teachers and friends left me exhausted and scarred inwardly – and occasionally outwardly!

Previous havens of security and warmth now caused me embarrassment and discomfort. My local church, which had been my extended family ever since I could remember, left me cold and alone. The Carol Service, in which I had once stood proudly as a red kilted angel, presented questions I couldn't answer. 'Unto you is born this day in the city of David, a Saviour which is Christ the Lord'. My voice had echoed confidently around the church on Christmas Eve. It was the last phrase of the angel's message that was the root of all my unrest, 'Christ the Lord'. Through my early years the name uppermost in my mind had been Sue and everything revolved around me. Now another name was competing for my attention. I tried to avoid it, ignore it, forget it. Its familiarity had been with me since birth. I had heard it in hymns, prayers and in conversations, frequently. Why now should it cause such confusion?

Thirty years on it would be easy to explain away the discomfort of those stumbling years, but thirty years on I remember a very similar confusion I felt when I was three years old. Daddy had also been a name I was familiar with. A day didn't pass without him being mentioned by a family who loved and missed him. The confusion came when, as a toddler, I discovered he was more than a name, more than a black and white photo. He was a strapping six footer who said he loved me and demanded a place in my life and our home. It took time to get to know him, to trust him, to accept his love and discipline. Then came the day in the tossing sea at Brighton. I was swung onto his broad shoulders and he started to swim out beyond the safety of the beach. I was petrified and clung to his strong back for dear life! This was my Dad and I needed him desperately. His knowledge of the sea and his physical strength carried me whimpering to safety.

Entering my teens caused a breaking away from the security of family life. It was like swimming out from the safety of the beach and riding the more powerful breakers of life. I had to grow up. I couldn't always play in the shallows. Outwardly life was full of excitement and promise. Inwardly I was afraid. Could I cope alone? For me to admit the need for outside help in life was hard. I was, and still am, a competitor, a fighter, I want to go it alone, I wouldn't be beaten!

With the growing battle came the growing awareness that Jesus, like my father, was more than just a name, more than a baby in a manger. I had heard all about him, but was it possible I could meet him and know him personally? Now each time I pushed his name aside it was rejection of a real live person, and the battle became more painful. Then came the day I met Jesus face to face! Nothing outwardly spectacular. Just a sudden, quiet recognition. All I had read, heard, and imagined came to three-dimensional life in a vivacious young woman, who had proved what she preached. She literally introduced me to Jesus, by showing him to me. I don't remember her words but her face revealed the answers to all my questions! Jesus is alive! He is real! I could know him personally!

This lady was no loser! Neither was she a robot! As a typical teenager, I had been afraid to lose my individuality, my independence. To ask God into my life surely meant admitting defeat, throwing in the towel. Suddenly here was a challenge. Should I face up to life and finally admit I couldn't cope? One of the strongest character building lessons in life is to admit failure and learn from it. In games I was constantly reminded 'If you can't cope with failure you will never handle success, you have to lose to win'. Was this the secret? In admitting my weakness could God make me strong? In recognizing my pride and selfishness could God change my attitude? After living several years of physical life, could he give me spiritual life?

The only way to find out was to put a verse I knew from the Bible to the test:

Listen! I stand at the door and knock. . .

I suddenly realized how that gentle knock had been disrupting my life recently.

If anyone hears my voice. . .

Light was dawning. The name of Jesus through my early years had become a persistent voice challenging me to action. Could that voice be God himself?

Hears my voice and opens the door. . .

The months of struggling against this unknown person melted away as I recognized the truth. It was up to me to stop fighting and open up the door of my life. A simple childlike step, but in that moment and ever since, I have experienced that God always keeps his promises.

I will come in (Rev 3:20 GNB).

Just as I received physical life in 1942, so in that moment in my teen years I received spiritual life. The battle in real life had only just begun!

3

FIT TO GROW

Gaining two-and-a-half stone in less than a year had its problems. In a matter of months I shot up to eleven stone and adjustments had to be made in clothing and occupation. From being a very active teacher, I became a very expectant Mum and was relieved when Stephen arrived healthy and whole, prompt at mid-day without one meal missed! I was drowsily fascinated as I watched the midwife weighing and measuring our little bundle of squalling humanity. That precious armful of baby, weighing eight pounds four ounces and measuring just twenty inches, is now studying for his 'A' levels and weighs in at ten-and-a-half stones and stands five feet eleven tall. Writing these inadequate words emphasizes the miracle that has taken place in our son over the last eighteen years. The miracle of growth!

Those tiny clenched fingers now stretch expertly over piano keys and guitar strings. The curled toes now pound tirelessly over football pitches, and those fragile arms, that I could encircle with finger and thumb, can now lift me effortlessly! The silent intricate processes of digestion, absorption, and metabolism mean very little to the vast majority of people. Yet without this invisible army of internal action, Stephen would not have survived. These incredible processes would also have been rendered useless without food. His physical growth and ability was and is dependent on the food he eats, and how he uses the energy produced from it.

From the day Stephen was born, his food has been used in three ways. It is either oxidized to produce energy for work and play; it is incorporated into new cells and tissues to produce growth; and it renews and replaces parts of tissue that are constantly being broken down by the chemical changes that occur during his life.

Until recently, I had never enjoyed being trapped at a desk writing. I found the process of learning slow and boring, and I longed to escape from the classroom and be free of books, diagrams and timetables. It was biology that started to capture my imagination. As students, we transformed the dull revision of physiology into colourful dramas, likening the journey of food through the digestive system to a western film. It was attacked at various passes, one being 'the duodenal pass', by juicy Indian characters from the 'Pancreas'! Amongst these were shady alkaline riders such as 'Trypsin'. The fun approach to study helped me with the struggle to absorb the basic facts about food and growth.

Our lack of understanding of anatomy and physiology does not change the fact that for steady growth and continuing health, a balanced diet of proteins, carbohydrates, fats, mineral salts, vitamins, water and roughage is essential. In our western society we have an abundance of aids to help us slim, trim or build. However in my distant days of study, it was very evident that a sensible balanced eating pattern should be an enjoyable disciplined way of life, rather than an occasional fad, or springtime expense.

As Stephen progressed from a noisily satisfying diet of milk, taken morning, noon and night, to minced vegetables, meat and porridge, his pattern of growth was very noticeable. From lazing and sleeping all day, he became alert and very much alive and kicking. All parents note with satisfaction and excitement, the obvious signposts of growth and development. The first smile, the first tooth, the first step and the first word. Later comes the first day at school, the first goal, or the first piano lesson. However, not once did I excitedly greet Doug, my husband, with 'he's digested his liver and bacon!' or 'the proteins from his boiled egg are building strong teeth and bones!' Yet without this unseen, unspectacular side of eating, none of those 'firsts' in growth would have been possible.

We have long since left the kitchen, where the faint pencil marks record the steady growth of two lively youngsters. For Duncan, our second son, it was one of the few unusual moments of breathless silence, as ceremoniously the pencil rested on his tousled head. The resulting yells of triumph echo in my memory as he discovered his creeping progress towards his goal. In his limited world, Stephen was the height of maturity, and he loved him. The nearer his faint dot crept to Stephen's height, the happier he was. One cold, bleak night, I was called desperately into his bedroom, by the words 'Mum, I've stopped growing!' In the darkness Duncan had started, perhaps for the first time, to grapple with the miracle of growth. We switched on the bedside light and I produced a large box of photographs. One by one he recognized a smaller, shorter Duncan, and he was able to compare his present size with that of a few years back. Photographs of his Dad when he was Duncan's age followed. He was both intrigued and fascinated as he enquired,

'Will I be as big as Dad one day!'

The sleepy son who turned over, happy with the prospect of future heights of stature, has in the past ten years or so, not only caught up with his big brother, but has left his Dad behind! It has however taken three solid meals a day over those years to keep that 'skin stretched over an appetite' growing!

It is sad that we lose sight of the miracle of physical growth with the passing years. The miracle becomes a battle in the western world against unwanted weight and extra inches. A balanced diet is even more necessary to maintain an ideal weight, for renewal of dying cells and tissue, and to produce energy for coping with life, whether it be heavy manual work, raising a family, or studying. The struggle however is deeper. As we diet, exercise or just joyfully ignore our expanding waistline, our battle goes beyond calories. It is against life itself, or the deterioration that physical life inevitably brings.

Joy taught me so much in the closing moments of her physical life. As the process of deterioration accelerated before my eyes, the sheer futility of physical life on its own hit me with brutal force. The excitement of birth, the years of growth and development, the laughter were drowned by the inevitability of death and decay.

The life that Jesus brings does not deteriorate or decay. Instead of destruction and death there is resurrection and life. Excitement and hope replace doom and despair. This was the living spiritual strength in Joy that grew and endured the most trying physical exhaustion. I shared in a miracle of spiritual growth against the dark backcloth of death.

Browsing through a bookshop recently, I discovered a section packed with books of all colours, shapes and sizes. Most of their introductions promised that the author could guarantee that the diet and way of life contained within their pages would introduce the reader to a new slimmer, healthier 'you'! The adjoining shelves were packed with a sedate stock of Bibles. As I compared the content of the two seemingly contrasting books, an intriguing similarity emerged. The author of the second book is God himself. There is only one Bible, even though it is printed in several translations and paraphrases. God's personal letter and communication to us contains his introduction, through his Son Jesus, to an entirely new life for each one of us. In 2 Corinthians 5:17 God says:

> When anyone is joined to Christ, he is a new being; the old is gone, the new has come (GNB).

Just as the other books further along the shelf proposed numerous diets, God not only introduces us to this new life, he also supplies the perfect balanced diet for growth. A diet that builds and strengthens our faith, releases energy for sharing it, and renews our spiritual life daily. Without this daily discipline of taking in and absorbing God's word, our lessons from physical growth make the outcome blatantly obvious. Our prayer life becomes paralysed, our faith falters, our communication collapses. The stunted growth in the lives of those in countries where they lack food is heartrending. The sadness that accompanies diseases such as anorexia nervosa emphasizes the spiritual tragedy of countries with millions of Bibles lying on shelves collecting dust, whilst underfed wilting Christians wonder why they are so ineffective. By listening to what God has to say to us through reading his word we are literally feeding spiritually. The Old Testament prophet Jeremiah said,

> When your words came, I ate them; they were my joy and my heart's delight (Jer 15:16)

and King David said,

Taste and see that the Lord is good (Ps 34:8).

An ideal taster for those approaching the Bible for the first time is the first four books of the New Testament. The gospels Matthew, Mark, Luke and John describe those years when Jesus himself lived on this earth. His life unfolds before us as seen through four pairs of eyes, which in his last three years followed his life and teaching. This starter can be supplemented with helpful booklets and explanatory notes such as:

1. *Every Day with Jesus* Special Edition for new Christians, by Selwyn Hughes (published by Crusade for World Revival).
2. *Young People's Every Day with Jesus* Also by Selwyn Hughes (Crusade for World Revival).
3. *Read, Mark, Learn* by John Blanchard (Henry Walter).
4. *Come Alive to God* for new Christians: God's word for today (Scripture Union).
5. *The Bible* by John Eddison (Scripture Union 1984).
6. *Listening to God* series edited by Martin Manser (Creative Publishing).
7. *Understanding the Bible* by John Stott (Scripture Union 1972).

One of the favourite meals in our family is a good, hot curry. The first taste is never sufficient. Silence descends as each delicious mouthful is chewed and swallowed. In the same way, as we discover that Jesus was not only a historical figure who died, but a living person who can relate to us, and live in us by his Holy Spirit, our diet must of necessity progress from simple tasters to more deeply satisfying meals. I remember with clarity the hunger cry of a newborn baby. The milk that so satisfied him in those early months is the ideal food, providing proteins, fats, carbohydrates, mineral salts and vitamins. All this goodness served in an easily absorbed liquid for the digestive system of the new arrival. Peter tells us

> Like newborn babies, crave pure spiritual milk, so that by it you may grow up in your salvation, now that you have tasted that the Lord is good (1 Pet 2:2-3).

In the Bible there is the complete nutritious food for new Christians accompanied by meaty chunks for maturing Christians. For adults the diet of milk is not satisfactory, owing to its high water content and lack of iron. In order for new babies to grow and become adults they must progress from milk to a varied diet of solids. The same is true of spiritual growth. To mature and grow strong and effective as God's children, we must feed progressively and solidly on God's word.

For many years I struggled to make the transition from that easy inadequate diet of milk of my early years in Bible reading. I knew the basics, but my Christian life cried out long and loud in its inadequacy for deep solid feeding on God's word. I lacked motivation and desire for further teaching and the years crept by as I picked and played with various verses of scripture. I looked upon reading the Bible as a drag and a bore and had no hunger for God's food. Like a physical baby I just automatically accepted what was fed to me, long into my teens. I was just existing spiritually on a spoon-fed diet of bits and pieces.

One of the stages of development in toddlers that can be the most frustrating is the messy, early attempts at feeding themselves. The spoon is rotated in all directions and the food sprayed everywhere but into the mouth. There is no clean, short cut in this learning process. The more they are encouraged to feed themselves the more skilful they become. The happier parents and toddler stay through this mucky stage the faster both parties develop in relationships, patience and feeding together.

After many years at playing around at reading the Bible, I discovered in John 16 verse 13 the words:

The Holy Spirit will guide you into all truth.

God the Holy Spirit is literally someone who comes alongside to guide and help. That new life conceived by the Holy Spirit in me could quietly develop and grow, not through my desperate efforts but through the continuing work of the Holy Spirit. We have a provider who is infinitely patient when we make a mess of spiritual feeding. He mops up the mess and breaks down the bread of life to enable us to digest, absorb and grow. My Bible lay open at John 16, when I realized, after much striving on my own, that I had never once asked God to give me a hunger for his word. Never had I asked him to guide and teach me the excitement of day-to-day living controlled by the Holy Spirit. My prayers consisted of uncertain requests ending with the words 'if it is your will', but I'd never thought of asking for those obvious gifts that God longs for his children to have.

'I just couldn't put it down.' How many times do we hear this said of a gripping novel, magazine or biography? God longs to give us the same absorption with the Bible if only we come as children and ask him. The soothing diet of milk drunk hungrily by small babies needs no teeth to start the process of digestion. Swallowed easily, it is smoothly digested and its goodness circulated throughout the body. To tackle the more substantial foods containing vital body-building ingredients, a strong set of teeth needs to cut those tiny gums. The growing child needs to learn to chew over and take time in eating richer solid foods.

As God increases our hunger for his word, we need to spend more time in cutting our spiritual teeth and chewing over what God has to say to us. Meditation causes apprehension amongst some Christians. Some associate it with academics while others connect it with the dangerous emptying of the mind as practised in some cults. Meditation on the Bible is in fact exercising the mind, not emptying it.

One of the ways I practise spiritual meditation, or chewing, is to take a verse or even a phrase that has challenged me from my daily reading. I memorize it and take it into the day with me. Just like the cow regurgitates food and chews it over, so I ask God to bring back to my memory those words, so that the Holy Spirit can apply them in the day's situations. With a laden trolley, I joined what seemed to be an endless stream to the cash desk. Perspiring mums grappled with tireless children, men signed cheques with sighs and the cashier wilted visibly as a very irate lady held everyone up with her selfish complaints. I was chewing over a verse early in Colossians chapter three and was in full, impatient flight:

Therefore, as God's chosen people . . . (v.12).

Tempers were rising as the complaints continued, when the following words pounded in my heart instead of in my head:

26

Bear with each other and forgive whatever grievances you may have against one another. Forgive as the Lord forgave you (v.13).

In a flash the Holy Spirit taught me to see that queue as God sees them. People he loves individually and has infinite patience with, and I was part of that queue!

Later on in that letter to the Colossians come the words:

Let the word of Christ dwell in you richly . . . (Col 3:16).

To allow the rich nutrition of God to saturate and permeate our lives, memorizing is essential. Again let us ask God to help us. The more we exercise our memories the more efficient they will be. As in physical exercise, start gradually and build up your capacity for memorizing. As our bodies shape up after continual physical exercise, so the spiritual exercises of memorizing and meditation will shape our thoughts and attitudes, our motives and desires. As memories are an intricate part of our human physical bodies they are naturally prone to deterioration for we become lazy in mind as well as body. Sluggishness in these areas will affect our spiritual lives. As we take note of our physical fitness, let us not forget the limbering up in our mental and spiritual lives that God can use to enable us to live to the full.

In Luke we read of someone who had perfect, all-round fitness.

Jesus grew in wisdom and stature, and in favour with God and men (Lk 2:52).

Through accepting God's answer in his Son Jesus to our human weakness and failure, God through his Holy

Spirit gives us the capacity for all-round fitness as seen in Jesus who lived that completely fit life on this earth.

'I doubt whether I'll ever keep it up' is a regular greeting I have from newcomers to our keep fit class in our church. Some have preconceived ideas as to what a keep fit class does, but few realize that as well as it being hard work we all enjoy ourselves so much. We might not feel like it at the start of the evening, but by the end we are relaxed and raring to go. Too often we approach the Bible not expecting to enjoy it. We open it in a cold academic light and forget that God is longing to speak right into our situation through it. This makes every approach to God's word an adventure.

An essential part of growth is not only building bones, muscles and tendons, but building up that vital resistance against germs that attack through the blood stream. The white cells in our blood ingest and destroy bacteria and dead cells by flowing round, engulfing and digesting them. The microscopic drama at the scene of a wound beats any up-to-date battle film. The white cells converge on the site of an injury or infection, and devour invading bacteria and damaged tissue. As a result they prevent the spread of harmful bacteria as well as accelerating the healing of the infected area. This process of protection is less effective without a balanced diet.

As we feed on God's word, not only is our faith built up, but our resistance and sensitivity to evil grows. The battering we take in life itself, which wounds and bruises our spirit is bathed by the soothing protection of his healing touch.

'To be of any value to the body, food taken in through the mouth must enter the blood stream and be distributed to all living regions.' Similar paragraphs can be found in the introduction to any chapter based on food and digestion in school textbooks. I longed at one time to write such an introduction for the spiritual food of the Bible, emphasizing the importance of taking in the words through our eyes, ears and minds and allowing the Holy Spirit to circulate and distribute it to all areas of our lives. I have discovered, however, that the most effective introductory paragraph is the irresistible life of the man or woman, boy or girl, who feeds long and hungrily on the word of God and increases the spiritual appetite of all those who come into contact with them.

We all know the famous words of 'Food Glorious Food' written by Lionel Bart for his musical *Oliver* based on Dickens' novel, *Oliver Twist*. The rough hungry days of the workhouse were brought to life again a few years back by our boys at their school. Parents thoroughly enjoyed the performances but this song was the highlight. The lack of good solid food causes the lads' imaginations to run riot and Lionel Bart captures their craving in this simple but powerful song. Part of our enjoyment was seeing our well-nourished teenagers singing of days they would never have to experience and yet in the twentieth century there is an appalling neglect of our spiritual diet. It is not only the youngsters who crave for a deeper, more satisfying life of meaning and purpose. A variety of diets can feed our minds and hearts causing us to grow up grotesque, handicapped, imbalanced. Sexual indulgence, love of material possessions, drug abuse are just some of those blatantly advertised in the twentieth-century menu.

The only diet which will bring balance, satisfaction and healthy growth in all areas is God's diet, contained in the Bible. Bibles, Christian books and helpful literature are in abundant supply in the west. We don't have to picture them or use our imaginations, as in some countries. Let's take the opportunity while we still have it, get out our Bibles, open them and allow God to feed us.

Psalm 36 verses 8-9 says:

We feast on the abundant food you provide; you let us drink from the river of your goodness. You are the source of all life! (GNB)

4

FIT FOR PRAYER

Our Christmas had been a good one. There had been time for family, friends, conversation, leisurely meals and moments to catch our breath after an eventful year. The early days of the New Year saw our home return to some form of normality and brought the first visit of the dustman. I handed him one last sack of rubbish and turned to enter my strangely bare hall, stripped of decorations and holly. The dustman called out to me,

'Hey love! Shall I take those?'

He was pointing to the two sprigs of artificial holly and a lonely Christmas rose lying on the doormat.

'No!' I laughed. 'They're not real—I might need them next year!'

That Christmas spray is etched on my memory and the seemingly insignificant conversation with a friendly refuse collector keeps echoing in my mind.

I am reminded of how prayer used to be. It looked effective enough. I used it for a while, then either discarded it, or packed it away, in case I might need it again, in the future. The fact of prayer was familiar to me. It cropped up on occasions, like holly at Christmas and then was forgotten. I went through the motions, learned from a loving family, and in my early teens came to know Jesus personally. But my prayers stayed in the parrot fashion style of childhood. Too often prayer lay discarded and lifeless on the doormat of my life. As a baby has to grow physically and learn how to communicate with its father and mother, so we must grow spiritually and learn to communicate with our heavenly Father. We must progress from those initial infant cries for attention if we are to experience the excitement and adventure of a continuous, two-way, living conversation and relationship with God.

How have Stephen and Duncan, my two teenage sons, acquired adult conversation that on occasions leaves me speechless? Through a continuously developing relationship with their parents. In their early years they were always with me. I cuddled them, talked to them, laughed with them and at times scolded them. My evangelist husband, Doug, was frequently away on missions so I shared everything with them. This resulted in my discovering how much a child responds to and is capable of communication. God is just longing to show us how much we are capable of by his Holy Spirit in and through prayer. As an ordinary Mum I lack maturity of judgement and wisdom, at times, in talking with my teenagers, but in prayer we have a Father who has perfect wisdom, patience and understanding. The more we spend time with him the more we will know prayer as an ongoing experience.

Many years ago I read these words by E. M. Bounds (in his book *Power through Prayer*): 'Prayer is a way of life, life is a way of prayer.' They are now becoming a living reality as I am learning that prayer is an attitude of life as well as special daily acts in my life.

The disciples who spent so much time with Jesus on this earth saw the power and impact of his perfect life. It was dynamite! As a result did they ask him for training in preaching techniques with the masses, in storm control on Galilee, in healing the sick? No! As they quietly observed his life, they pinpointed the source, and said:

Lord, teach us to pray (Lk 11:1).

That simple request led to teaching about prayer, that equipped the disciples for a tough future, when without communication with God they would have collapsed. It has held the key right down through the centuries to living life to the full with continual consultation with the Person who gave us life in the first place. He knows our limitations and frustrations and can help us cope with them. He sees our potential and wants to fulfil it in us. My discovery of prayer as a vital experience grew from my joining the ranks of those disciples who have echoed those words personally:

Lord teach me to pray.

I am being led into four basic areas of practice, although I have known the theory for years. Firstly, *be simple*. This shouldn't be too hard a lesson to learn. But what a tangled web we weave in prayer! My motives, attitudes, hopes and fears can all complicate my approach to God. Words that help me are:

Jesus take me as I am,
I can come no other way.
Take me deeper into You,
Make my flesh life melt away.
Make me like a precious stone,
Crystal clear and finely honed.
Life of Jesus shining through,
Giving glory back to You.
Dave Bryant, © Thankyou Music 1978.

I need to be honest and straightforward in my approach to God and expect answers. That 'fine honing' can be painful but is so necessary! I am learning not to beat about the bush and to come straight to the point. It is such a shame that so often only pain, tragedy or disaster brings the directness in prayer that God longs for.

At the age of six, I thought that the height of maturity was to stand at the ironing board and press the creases out of a mountain of washing. Today a basket full of shirts turns that dream into a nightmare! How I longed in those early days to iron the handkerchieves. The opportunity came and my mother left me in charge. I finished the neat pile of linen and with great care unplugged the iron and stood it to cool. Having reached maturity, I decided to continue in my mother's footsteps in swiftly banging the board into its folded position. I had admired her dexterity in this glorious thumping event and couldn't wait to 'have a go'. My six-year-old fingers were placed at one end, and then, slightly tilting the board, I gave the other end a tremendous thump! I remember to this day the pain that followed. The heavy old board crushed my fingers, and all I could do was literally gasp for help—a simple cry of agony!! My mother heard it and hurtled downstairs to release me. The original meaning of Hebrews 2 verse 18 is God is able to run to the cry of his children. I am slowly learning to be as simple and direct in my appreciation, praise and confession as I am in my urgent cries for help.

My childhood prayers were regularly closed with 'God bless all the people all over the world, and Timmy the cat!' I was specific enough about the cat who mattered to me, but the rest of the world was beyond my comprehension. God gives attention to detail. He knows my name (Is 43:1), and every facet of my nature (Jer 1:5).

I need to take time to get to know him so I can *be specific* in my praise of who he is as well as what he does

(Ps 103). When vagueness creeps into prayer, it paralyses it. Just as 'world' in my childhood prayers covered a multitude of people, so the word 'sin' covers literally a multitude of sins. I need the discipline of keeping short accounts and confessing specific sins so that God can cleanse my mind and heart. Any fuzziness in the use of the word 'sin' can lead to unconfessed hurt, misunderstanding, and bitterness. I am continually challenged by a translation, from the Chinese, of Psalm 139 verses 23-24:

> Oh God examine me (as in the customs). Test my inmost thoughts, intentions and meanings. Look right inside me (X-ray me) and see if there is hate, evil in my being. You may take my hand along the Heavenly way.

Taking this as my own prayer, I wrote down those inmost thoughts, intentions and meanings. The X-ray eye of God rooted out the specific hate and evil and confronted by them in cold print, I realized afresh the gift of forgiveness. After confessing each specific sin I determined that tearing up that sheet of paper was not sufficient. I burnt it and rejoiced that God remembers those sins no more.

To be specific in prayer I have developed a weekly prayer diary. Each page is headed with the day of the week and contains the names of people and the situations that I am committed to pray for regularly. As items arise for prayer, I add them to the appropriate day with comments when God answers prayer. To look back over that diary is a constant encouragement and raises the expectation level of my faith as I see what God has done in lives and circumstances.

Activity and impulsiveness are marks of my character and to sit for any length of time capturing my thoughts on paper is difficult. The other day as I was working on this chapter, I dropped everything and on the spur of the moment headed for the beach and the pounding surf to catch a breath of fresh air. It is said that we can speak to God at any time or place, but do we take advantage of this exceptional spiritual gift? God is teaching me through my impulsive nature, not only to be disciplined in prayer but also to *be spontaneous* in prayer. To use those sudden times of needed change to gain fresh opportunities for speaking with him, helping me to have an awareness of God in all my situations. As I walked, dodging the spray tossed up by the windswept sea, I filled my lungs with clean, salty air. The sharp breeze cleared my mind, and my muddled thoughts started tumbling out to the one person who understands me completely. Ahead the coast swept on to Poole, and Swanage faded in the storm clouds—and there was not a soul in sight. But I wasn't alone. Just as Jesus walked by the sea with his disciples, so he walked with me listening to my hopes, fears and concerns. There is a time for systematic communication with God, but if I always waited until I am organized, I would never make it! We don't tell our children not to talk to us until they are grammatically perfect in their English. Their verbal stumblings are interpreted by a loving and understanding parent who is delighted by the fragile attempt at communication because it enables a relationship to be developed and deepened. God understands our varying temperaments and weaknesses and longs to hear from us however we feel. Those walks by the sea are a 'breath of fresh air' to my mind, body and spirit. Here I can freely share with God those things that are on my heart. Without interruption I voice my thoughts and sing those hymns and choruses that are direct prayers.

I love you Lord, and I lift my voice,
To worship you, O my soul rejoice!
Take joy my King in what you hear,
Let it be a sweet, sweet sound in your ear.

Mingled with the roar of the wind and thunder of the sea my voice is not drowned out because God longs to hear from me his child!

Having company on a long car journey helps time to pass quickly and interesting conversation keeps me alert and improves my concentration. I seem to be spending more and more time driving and find it a valuable opportunity to pray and great for spontaneity in sharing with God. Travelling through hills, villages or towns, God uses the kaleidoscope of life I am seeing to spur me on to pray. Stopping for children, racing for school, reminds me of those I know at home concerned for exams or football matches, teachers and students. An ambulance, the postman, birds following a lone tractor, or roadworks all can trigger off a train of thought which becomes prayer when shared aloud or silently with my unseen passenger. I love starting the day driving through darkened silent roads, as the sun rises and the traffic multiplies. The wakening world whether crisp with frost or drenched with rain speaks of God's love and care and can draw from my heart spontaneous thanks and praise.

Much of my childhood was spent standing on my head! I could never sit still or wait patiently. With exception to the headstands, this still holds true. I would rather 'get up and go' than observe from the sidelines. My son Duncan has inherited this tendency. Fourteen years ago it was his first visit to the dentist. It is still very clear in my memory. The dentist was extremely patient and understanding as he built up the toddler's confidence in him. The dental chair became an aeroplane and Duncan pressed every button in sight. Different-sounding instruments were put into action and multi-coloured mouthwashes sampled. As the two-year-old grew weary, he sank back into the leather chair. With a sigh of relief, the dentist said,

'O.K., son. Let's be still. Open up and I'll take care of those teeth.'

I have discovered that my spontaneity in prayer, if not controlled by God, can lead to a frantic striving to solve the problems myself. Just as Duncan had to be still to allow the expert to deal with the problem tooth, so I am learning to *be still* in God's company. To enjoy his presence and listen to his voice. To open up my life for his touch of encouragement, correction or challenge. Many of the 'gods' worshipped today from popstars to sportsmen welcome plenty of noise and applause in adoration of them. As the screaming mounts and the drums roll I am reminded of the contrasting entrance God made to this world, clothed as man in Christ Jesus. Throughout his comparatively short life on this earth, he frequently shrank from the crowds and the attention of his followers to spend time alone in communication with his Father. His disciples were encouraged in the same practice when he invited them to join him:

Come with me by yourselves to a quiet place and get some rest. (Mk 6:31)

In my crowded day-to-day living I am learning to answer swiftly that command:

Be still, and know that I am God (Ps 46:10).

I have built more deep, lasting relationships in our

Church Keep Fit group in the last five years than at any other time in my life. We enjoy the sixty minutes of exercise but it is interesting to note that the most difficult exercise for most people is to relax and be still. It has to be worked at and practised. The same goes for that spiritual stillness which will always lead to more effective action.

From the words preceding Psalm 46 verse 10, I can see why the Good News version says:

Stop fighting . . . and know that I am God.

The prayer that changed the whole direction of my life in my early teens was stark in its simplicity! I don't remember the words—I just remember a 'Cease Fire!' God said 'stop fighting' and I did. In the stillness, I knew he had come into my life.

The years passed and I stood at the kitchen sink elbow deep in soap suds and nappies. My two boys were sleeping. As I stood looking across the toy-strewn lawn, I poured out my pent-up feelings to God who had stuck with me through thick and thin! I felt tired, inadequate and useless. Again God spoke through that verse—'Be still, stop fighting!' My struggle was with the mundane tasks which seemed never ending. I was kicking against domesticity and feeling hopelessly trapped. The words first spoken to the blind man in Luke 18 verse 40, God now spoke right into my kitchen:

What do you want me to do for you? (GNB)

Like a child, I didn't really know, and I told him so.

'I just want to be useful, please show me what I can do.'

In direct answer to that prayer God took the very home and circumstances in which I felt so stifled and exhausted and opened it up for fresh opportunities in introducing friends and neighbours to the personal God I had met so many years before.

Prayer is an individual, personal experience and one prayer often on my lips and in my heart today is expressed in words written by Graham Kendrick.

Restore O Lord
The honour of your name.
In works of sovereign power
Come shake the earth again,
That men may see
And come with reverent fear
To the living God,
Whose kingdom shall outlast the years.

Graham Kendrick & Chris Robinson, © Thankyou Music 1981.

If God is to answer this prayer we have to stop our fighting and allow God to make us fit for action. It is his action that is so effective.

5

FIT FOR ACTION

The two weeks of Wimbledon are full of thrills and spills. Crowds cheer and groan as their eyes swing from end to end of the tramlined rectangle called a tennis court. From America to Australia, Czechoslovakia to Chile, top tennis players come to pit their skills and fitness against fellow competitors. The arrogant power of champions is challenged by the impudent freshness of newcomers. One thing is certain, that to win, each player must be totally and systematically prepared physically and mentally for each match. Reaching their peak in fitness, skill and mental alertness takes total dedication and determination.

From Wimbledon to Wembley, in Vietnam or the Falklands, in sport and war, wherever there is action, there is a need for preparation and fitness. Directly the Task Force received their orders to proceed to the Falklands, the men were training on board ship, preparing for the specific task that lay ahead. The success of their action in those islands lay in their training and preparation.

Another urgent call for action has echoed through the centuries. The command of God is 'Go!' Not only to the Falklands, but to the whole world! There is a desperate need for the good news of Jesus to be proclaimed and experienced on every continent, in every country, town, village, street, home and family. God is enlisting a task force for action. He is building a people of power. He is not interested in immobile, complacent, overweight Christians taking in his truth all the time, and never working it out in practice. Jesus said 'Be ye doers of the word and not hearers only' (Jas 1:22 AV). Let's start our spiritual work-out session right here. God isn't feeding us from his word to make spiritually obese believers. He builds us for action. He reaches the world through his people. Duncan Campbell said:

> What the world needs to see is the wonder and beauty of God-possessed personalities, men and women with the life of God pulsating within, who practise the presence of God and consequently make it easy for others to believe in God.
>
> (Quoted in David Watson, *I Believe in the Church*, Hodder & Stoughton 1978.)

Before we are tempted to 'do a Jonah', and run in the opposite direction, let's remember that God doesn't leave us out on a limb. Linked with the call to 'Go' is the promise 'I will be with you always' (Mt 28:20). God does not mock us. He never calls us to a task without giving the power to fulfil it. Melody Green wrote these words:

> Thank you O my Father for giving us your Son,
> And leaving your Spirit till the work on earth is done.
>
> From Melody Green, *There is a Redeemer*, copyright © 1982 Birdwing/Word Music (UK), a division of Word (UK) Ltd, Northbridge Road, Berkhamsted, Herts HP4 1EH, England. Used by permission.

When the crunch comes the lone Channel swimmer or the Wimbledon finalist must go it alone. They rely on all the months of preparation and training leading up to the event. No one else can swim those gruelling miles, or walk out onto that electrifying Centre Court. In contrast when God says 'Go!', he launches out with us, whether to other countries, or across the street, into the office, factory, school or home. He puts his limitless resources at our disposal. He goes ahead of us and works at both ends of the line. As we answer that call to 'Go', God replaces our inadequacies with his qualities and ability.

In working out our faith in daily witness, we need his power and strength flowing through us to others. This enables us to build relationships and earn the right to share naturally the marvellous piece of good news the world has never truly considered. Let's not waste time excusing our reluctance and bemoaning our spiritual deficiencies. Step out in faith and obey God's word, and discover how he has prepared us for the task. 'You did not choose me, but I chose you. . .(Jn 15:16).

When the lunchtime bell rang at my school, I was always the first to hurtle from the classroom into the playground. In my junior days it wasn't long before we were picking teams for our chosen game. I recollect clearly the sinking realization that everyone else was being chosen before me. Eventually all were included, but the feeling of rejection and being left out creeps into all our lives and leaves its mark. Whether we weren't chosen for the job we wanted, or by the partner we longed for, the sense of inadequacy eats away inside us. Take heart—Jesus says to us: 'Come on! Come and be in my team. I choose you. Not because I feel sorry for you—but because I love you, and need you. Without you, my task force is incomplete.' We are of value and worth to God. His chosen people. We might not feel very special. The danger is to be constantly comparing ourselves with others. We will always find someone more effective, better looking, and with a superior gift to us. God is less interested in our ability than in our availability to him. It's not our appearance but the reflection of his character in us that matters.

We are not only chosen people, but 'holy and dearly loved' also. 'Holy, holy, holy, Lord God Almighty' was a favourite hymn of mine at primary school. It led me, however, to understand that holiness was exclusively related to God's person and certainly had nothing to do with 'little old me'! I was too insignificant and useless to be considered 'holy'. I was therefore intrigued to find we are described as 'holy' in Colossians chapter 3 verse 12. Further study uncovered an exciting depth to this word. It means I could be set apart for a very special task. As God chose me, so he identified a specific work he has for me to do. That makes me special, and vital to the balance and efficiency of God's team.

Rugby, football, netball and hockey are all team games which need mature management, skilled coaching and wise guidance. The most successful teams have talented players who exhibit total confidence in their manager and trainer. The latter develops character as well as basic skills. Players are encouraged to reach their full potential and use it for the benefit of the team. To be fit for action in God's team we have at our disposal the finest manager and expert coach who not only has our peak performance at heart, but created every skill and gift in us. He has wisdom and perception in moulding and developing our obvious strengths and even uncovers hidden abilities. Before the match the team talk is essential and must be listened to carefully. Understanding what the manager wants can mean the difference between victory or failure. Our team talk is found in Colossians chapter 3 verses 12-17.

Firstly, we are to be a *prepared team*. 'Clothe yourselves,' he urges. Each sport requires individual clothing. To play an ice-hockey match in lightweight swimming trunks might give the player an edge in speed, but not in protection from the fierce tackles of the opposition. He'd soon be badly battered. The substantial padding and helmets are essential in this fast, tough sport. Because there is no short cut to introducing Jesus to friends and neighbours, all the advice about how to do it more efficiently should be carefully considered. Paul pleads,

> . . . clothe yourselves with compassion, kindness, humility, gentleness and patience. . .And over all these virtues put on love, which binds them all together in perfect unity (Col 3:12-14).

In recent years thousands of holidaymakers have made their way to the Royal Showground at Wadebridge in Cornwall. They participate in a special week for the family called Royal Week, sponsored by *Family* and *Buzz* magazines. As a family we have enjoyed attending this event, and been challenged and stimulated by the worship and teaching. After one evening meeting, my youngest son and I ran through the rain to our caravan. Hanging up our soaking clothes, we jumped into our sleeping bags. After an action-packed week, sleep wasn't far away, but on the fringe of my consciousness hovered the thought that the other members of the family, Doug and Stephen, would be equally tired and wet. For them to drip everywhere in a tiny caravan would cause havoc, so I needed to stop them in the doorway. The continual drum of rain on the caravan lulled me to sleep, when suddenly our caravan door crashed open. With eyes still closed I sat bolt upright in my sleeping bag and snapped, 'Stand there and strip off!' There was a stunned silence and slowly I opened my eyes. In the dim light of a gas mantle stood a complete stranger! His eyes had the expression of a startled rabbit. In the confusion of rain and darkness he had returned to the wrong caravan! Strangely, God used that hilarious occurrence to highlight the tragedy of attempting any action without the necessary spiritual clothing and preparation.

Dressing physically doesn't just happen. A daily routine is necessary. A simple snap of the fingers doesn't produce a 'Mary Poppins' style transformation, convenient as that would be! Similarly, it is a regular, hourly exercise to ask God to clothe us with his compassion, his kindness, his gentleness, his humility, his patience and his love. This clothing is for our protection, warmth and appearance, to help us draw alongside other people and show them the character of Jesus. These clothes never go out of fashion. Comparatively recent photos illustrate the vast changes in fashion, styles and colours and cause endless amusement to the young.

The compassion seen in Jesus weeping over Jerusalem; the kindness that produced the best festive wine in an emergency; the gentleness which forgave a sinner; the humility that stooped to wash the disciples' dirty feet; the patience that welcomed children when his friends tried to encourage solitude; and the love that cried in agony from the cross 'Father, forgive them, for they do not know what they are doing' (Lk 23:34) are all available to us today and will never go out of fashion with God.

As Paul continues to write or dictate this letter in a Roman prison, he tells us to be a *caring team*. Good relationships between players on the same side are crucial. Harmony and loyalty are essential to peak performance. To observe a well-balanced unit working together and supporting one another in defence and attack is great entertainment. In evangelism the love we have for one another must be visible. If relationships in and between churches and Christians are not right it doesn't speak much of our manager.

> Bear with each other and forgive whatever grievances you may have against one another. Forgive as the Lord forgave you (Col 3:13).

Jamie was just five years old and his prize possession was his train set. Returning home from school one day, he found that his little sister Heidi had smashed his favourite engine. What Jamie wasn't going to do to his sister was nobody's business! He was livid! He was going to bash her head in. Mum kept them apart for the rest of the day and with Heidi safely in her cot asleep, she went along to Jamie's room for prayer time. 'God bless Mummy, Daddy, Nanny, Grandpa, and all the Aunties and Uncles'—but there was no mention of Heidi. Mum explained to Jamie, as simply as she could, about loving and forgiving. But it didn't help, he was going to bash her head in. 'Jamie, just suppose you died tonight and had to meet God and you hadn't forgiven your sister. Do you think God would be pleased?' Jamie thought about it then he clenched his fists and closed his eyes. Taking a deep breath he said, 'God bless Heidi and I forgive her for damaging my train set. Amen. P.S. Dear God, if I don't die tonight I'm going to bash her head in in the morning!' We may smile at the transparency of a child. They are so open about their grudges which they quickly forget, but as we grow older we learn to hide our feelings. Our grudges are disguised but that unforgiving spirit is one of the main factors in the failure of the team. 'Forgive as the Lord forgave you' should be our team motto.

'Let the peace of Christ rule in your hearts. . . Let the

word of Christ dwell in you richly' (Col 3:15-16) are an encouragement to a *controlled team*. We must listen carefully to God's instructions and implement them. In my early days of hockey it was very hard to see the point of the game. Twenty-two pairs of legs all converged on one tiny ball. Sticks were not carried, they were brandished and both teams usually ended up in a collapsed heap in the goal-mouth. As the years passed and we listened to our games teacher, we learned the wisdom of making room for each other, of passing the ball well ahead for another forward to run into position, and in working up opportunities for others to score the goals. The work of salvation is not ours, it is God's, and we need to be controlled by him to reach those people he is preparing by his Holy Spirit. He says, 'Let the peace of Christ rule in your hearts, since as members of one body (one team) you were called to peace' (Col 3:15). Plastered over many walls in London are slogans such as 'Arsenal rules O.K.!' and 'Chelsea forever!' For our team to be effective, the word of God that endures forever needs to dwell in us and control us and the peace of Christ must rule!

A team that enjoys the game will work well together in spite of setbacks. But when the joy of playing is replaced by the love of money, performance is affected. God's team is the most exciting team to be in and he wants us to be a *cheerful team*. There is plenty to cheer about! 'As you sing psalms, hymns and spiritual songs with gratitude in your hearts to God' (Col 3:16). God longs for us to bring warmth and real cheer back into the hearts and lives of those around us. 'Joy is the serious business of heaven', said C. S. Lewis and it should be of earth also. Not a false jolliness that drives everyone up the wall, but the quiet contentment that Paul experienced in trials and difficulties that caused him to say, 'I have learned to be content whatever the circumstances' (Phil 4:11).

This powerful, pre-action talk in Colossians 3 nears its end with the words 'and whatever you do, whether in word or deed, do it all in the name of the Lord Jesus' (v. 17). It is his work. Philippians chapter 1 verse 6 reads 'Being confident of this, that he who began a good work in you will carry it on to completion.' A team is chosen for its various strengths and gifts. The goal-scoring skill of a forward is as important as the courage and consistency of a full back. No player is more important than another, although some are more noticeable. I long to give the lone 'goalie' a big hug after his side have scored and all attention is showered on his forwards. An essential part of the winning team, he often stands alone enjoying his team's success, yet without him the score would be very different. We all have vital gifts given to us by God that need to be developed and used.

Several Christmases ago my husband Doug gave me a very special present. He had taken great care and thought over it. Others might well have thought it comparatively small and uninteresting—even boring. Doug knew it was just what I wanted, and needed. The compact brown leather notebook has been with me ever since. The temptation, when given a precious gift, is to say 'thank you', wrap it up, and place it safely away. It is, however, the best silent thanks for Doug to see that notebook, several years later, packed with notes, the cover several shades lighter, slightly stained, but thoroughly used! We are to be a *charismatic team,* attracting others to the gospel by the quality of life they see in us. Let's use the obvious talents the Lord has given us and ask him what other gifts he has for us and needs to develop in us for the task ahead.

Every person I come into contact with reads a Bible!

Not the leather-bound edition but one that is covered in flesh. It is my Life Edition!

We are the only Bible a sinful world will read,
We are the sinner's gospel, we are the scoffer's creed,
We are the Lord's last message written in word and deed.
What if the type is crooked?
What if the print is blurred?
What if our hands are busy with work other than his?!

God gave me a final challenge as I considered the plans he has for his team. He gave me a glimpse of the team, when we are not submissive to his management and guidance. If we are not his *charismatic* team, using the gifts he has given us, then sadly we are *crippled* and never reach our full potential. If we are not his *cheerful* team, we are *choked* up with ourselves so that God cannot fill us with his revitalizing Spirit. Unless we are his *controlled* team we will be *careless* and thoughtless. His *caring* team will become *critical* and hurtful towards each other and all those they come into contact with. The absence of God's spiritual clothes will bring a chill to our approach and a cold aloofness will drive people away. If we haven't been chosen individually to be part of God's team, if we haven't accepted Jesus into our lives to start the coaching process that will make us more like him and ready for action, then the Bible tells us very clearly, we are condemned. God says in Romans 6 verse 23 'For the wages of sin is death. . .' But God never intended physical and spiritual death, for that verse continues: 'the gift of God is eternal life in Christ Jesus our Lord.' Receive the gift. Join the team and get into the action!

6

FIT TO DROP!

Despair and disbelief froze his features as he bent over his dying daughter. Just a few short minutes before, she had run excitedly into his surgery. Bubbling over with life and energy, the seven-year-old thrust a small jagged gash in front of the experienced eye of her father.

'A rusty nail did it Daddy!', she told him.

As a much loved and well-established doctor, her father had given numerous anti-tetanus injections. Tenderly he swung his only daughter onto his lap. She was the apple of his eye, arriving after three strapping sons, and his strong fingers gently tended the wound. The injection was hardly noticed by his trusting daughter and she lay back on the consulting room couch . . . where, minutes later, she died.

This was in 1956, before the days of the much safer Tetanus toxoid. The lively seven-year-old body suffered a massive anaphylatic reaction and nothing her father could do, completely single-handed, was of any avail. A telephone call to one of his colleagues was rapidly answered, but between them nothing could be done. The tragedy caused a wave of shock throughout the town: all the doctors admitted they would have done exactly the same for their daughters, and parents hugged their daughters and thanked God for them. I was just seven years older than my cousin when she died, and the wave of shock hit our family.

Twenty-eight years later my uncle wrote to me saying 'Only the Lord knows the results for eternity from this outward-looking tragedy. "In all things God works together for good to those who love Him" (Rom 8:28). At the time I was away from the Lord. The psalmist in Psalm 40 has just put words in my mouth, "He brought me out of the miry clay (he dragged me out by the scruff of my neck) and set my feet on a rock (that rock is Christ) and put a new song into my mouth." Since that day our family has been knit together as never before.'

In the twentieth century it is not only individuals who experience despair and disillusionment but villages, towns and nations. The whole world confronts disaster, violence, unemployment, war and disease and experiences the misery of defeat plus the fatigue of fighting such a wide variety of battles. It doesn't always take world shattering events to plunge us into gloom. Those seemingly insignificant mishaps can accumulate and drag us down physically, mentally and spiritually. After action of any description, we must expect to experience fatigue to some degree. Life itself exhausts and drains us but there are steps that can be taken to avoid destructive weariness and certainly the loss of heart that saps the energy and brings a sense of hopelessness and desolation.

Where can we turn when we are at the end of our tether and fit to drop? Various solutions are recommended! We may be ordered or urged to 'Snap out of it'. A talk with a psychiatrist or doctor could be a help. Changing our job and moving house can produce a temporary diversion, but these can present a whole new set of problems. Another holiday, a new romance, diet, outfit or makeup can all create fresh boosts to our ego, but the lasting answer does not lie here.

For times like these the answer is to be found in the word of God and the person it introduces us to, Jesus Christ. Instead of snapping out of it, we can get stuck into real living; instead of talking it through endlessly with specialists and friends, we can pray it through with the only expert on individual life; instead of getting away from it all, we can have peace within it all; instead of a new outfit, we can be an entirely new person—as we read in 2 Corinthians 5:17:

> Therefore, if anyone is in Christ, he is a new creation; the old has gone, the new has come!

Instead of a new fleeting romance, we can have a vital lasting relationship with Jesus himself, who picks us up, dusts us down, and gives us a fresh zest for living.

When we lose heart we lose sight of the central purpose of living crystallized in Ephesians 1 verses 11-12 as 'for the praise of his glory'. As we direct all our doubts and fears onto the one person who has been through our experience and never lost heart, we will be encouraged. Jesus knew weariness (Lk 8:23) and pain (Lk 22:63-65), but never fear or doubt. He experienced man's envy (Mt 27:18) and disloyalty (Mt 26:56), but through it all he never gave up. He *is* the life he offers. His endurance and encouragement must be lived out through me. He must be at the heart of every decision and be in the centre of every activity.

It had been a very long week with many late nights, plus the mental strain that accompanies a household where two teenagers are taking vital exams. I sat at my kitchen table with a coffee and my Bible open at Hebrews chapter 12. I was extremely weary and with the depressing comments resulting from the exams had lost heart several days before. I strove to take in the words that swam before my eyes, but my thoughts were elsewhere. The boys, their future, the dinner, all these fought for my attention, until a phrase literally jumped out at me!

. . . so that you will not grow weary and lose heart (v.3).

What had I missed? What was the prescription or tonic I had to take to prevent fatigue and desperation? I read through the previous three verses again and found three vital steps that, if followed, give us extra energy, stamina and challenge.

Firstly in verse 1 it says:

Let us throw off everything that hinders and the sin that so easily entangles.

To be a life saver in swimming, the student has to cover a certain distance in the water with his clothes on. You rapidly appreciate the handicap a skirt, trousers, blouse or shirt can be when you try to move through the water at speed. The blouse billows up round your face and hinders breathing and the trousers cling heavily to your legs. The relief is considerable when at the end of the ordeal, still treading water, the clothes can be peeled off and you complete the rest of the test unhindered. This freedom has to be experienced to be believed. Similarly much of the weariness and loss of heart in our Christian lives is due to the accumulated clutter that weighs us down and impedes progress. Wrong relationships, needless activity, inattention to prayer and Bible reading, poor personal discipline and slack attitudes are just a few hindrances that cause spiritual sluggishness and prevent us reaching a drowning world with God's salvation. It is not always the obvious things that entangle and crush our spiritual life, but the subtle intertwining of wrong motives, hidden thoughts and dubious desires.

My favourite fresh vegetable is the runner bean, especially if it is picked straight from the garden. Our first attempt at growing them was a fascinating experience for our young sons, each of whom had been allocated his own plant. The creeping progress of the new plants, as they wrapped their leaves round the lattice work of bean poles, intrigued them. To increase the interest, we challenged each other as to which plant would reach the top of its pole first. Slug pellets were scattered to protect them, and we carefully watered and sprayed them each night. It was some time before I noticed an almost identical plant steadily wrapping its shoots round the poles. It wasn't until the scarlet flower, forerunner of the bean, appeared that I discovered the interloper—commonly known as bindweed. No red flower or bean was forthcoming with this weed. It just strangled and stunted the growth of the real vegetable. The longer the bindweed was left, the more difficult it was to separate and release its tentacles from the plant, and unless it was completely uprooted it rapidly regrew to once again stifle the crop.

Many good and healthy pastimes can, if not guarded, subtly choke and drain that tender spiritual life growing within us. We must regularly bring all our activity to God, allowing him to root out any lethargy or destructive and restrictive practices that prevent us bearing Jesus' life fruit. A simple down-to-earth exercise I have found helpful is to take a sheet of paper and mark out three columns on it, headed:

1. Activities I want to do.
2. Activities others want me to do.
3. Activities God wants me to do.

The prayerful discipline of analysing our activities often reveals areas where we are not needed though still involved. Conversely it can show other activities that God is very clearly leading us into. This is not to infer that everything God wants us to do will be contrary to our personal desires. Nor does it imply that the pressure of Christian associates is always wrong. Truly there is real enjoyment in fulfilling God's plan for our lives, but those activities motivated solely by my selfish desire or the persuasion of friends and family should be carefully examined and questioned. Throwing off everything that hinders and the sin that entangles can be a lengthy and sometimes painful process. But it will always lead to a greater freedom and joy in our relationship with God and a greater effectiveness in our service for him.

Our second step is also discovered in verse 1. To build stamina and prevent weariness, we are told to 'run with perseverance the race marked out for us' (Heb 12:1).

A variety of races are included in the Olympic Games. Athletes train seriously and fight hard for their places in the national squad that will go to the Games. They know they will compete against some of the fastest men and women in the world. The most gruelling race has got to be the Marathon, stretching just over 26 miles.

There is, however, another and longer race that has obstacles and demands stamina. The Human Race! Without exception, we are all competitors in this event.

We set out alone but whether we experience the loneliness of the long distance runner, or ask for the company and help of someone who has pounded the track before us, is up to us. Jesus has competed in and victoriously completed the human race. He gloriously overcame the hopeless ending of death. He gives us his ability to run our individually marked out course. He knows what lies ahead and the energy we are going to require. His Holy Spirit supplies the power (Acts 1:8), control and thrust that is necessary for every bend and in every long straight. He gives the perseverance that overcomes the reckless impatience that causes us to run at top speed for a while but to drop out when the muscles tire; the tenacity that holds on when the crippling cramp of criticism knocks us down; the persistence that enables us to pull through when disappointment and failure dog our footsteps; and the steadfastness that sees us smoothly through the bad times as well as the good.

One of the toughest sections of the transatlantic single-handed yacht race, which covers the long route to Newport, Rhode Island, is when the boats hit headwinds without any protection from land. The force of these winds can add 800 miles to the race and more energy, hair, money and weight is lost than at any other time in the race, just struggling to keep going. It is no wonder that in the battle against life's strong winds of adversity, we grow weary and lose heart. As Christians, we can learn some interesting lessons from the way competitors prepare themselves for their activities.

A regular balanced diet is vital to build power for sudden bursts of explosive energy, or for prolonged bouts of sustained effort. In this day and age, with numerous aids to encourage Bible study, there is no excuse for us to starve spiritually. I find the wide variety of devotional cassette tapes provide a real ministry to me in my busy life. In my car, at my ironing board and in the garden, I can learn from leading Bible teachers. Invest in some of these and build yourself up so that you will have something to draw on in the demanding times of action.

Athletes must maintain a regular rhythm of breathing throughout the race. This enables the body to receive sufficient oxygen to fuel the effort required from heart, lungs and muscles. During our earthly race we must breathe deeply in prayer to our heavenly Father. It is vital that we cultivate a continual rhythm in our prayer life. This maintains our dependence upon the power that God provides through his Holy Spirit. Our own strength will fade and die but

> I can do all things in him who strengthens me (Phil 4:13 RSV).

Successful competitors go to bed early. They make sacrifices in their social life in order to get proper rest, then they can run relaxed. A considerable amount of our spiritual sluggishness could be remedied with a programme of regular sleep and relaxation. We are told that 'in quietness and trust is your strength' (Is 30:15) and in addition we are commanded to 'Be still and know that I am God' (Ps 46:10).

Systematic exercise, progressively building towards peak performance, is always in the mind of an athlete. He plans his training to reach prime performance at the race. God's instructions will keep us spiritually toned up.

Perseverance is encouraged by looking at previous champions and learning from their achievements and techniques. In Hebrews 11 we see God's gold medalists in the Olympic Games of Faith. Abraham kept running when he wasn't sure where God was leading him (Gen 12). Noah didn't lose heart even when he acted against popular opinion and built a gigantic boat with no water in sight (Gen 6). Moses held on in there, even though criticism came from the children of Israel and members of his own family (Num 12). But we look beyond these to Jesus himself 'who endured the cross, scorning its shame' and 'who endured such opposition' (Heb 12:2-3) and yet never lost heart.

Our third step is the most important:

Let us fix our eyes on Jesus (Heb 12:2)

Our younger son, Duncan, loves the game of rugby and played in the First Fifteen at school. He was introduced to rugby at junior school and grew to love the game. He loved the speed, the tackles; the supreme joy of scoring his first try is etched in my memory. He came into the house tired, dirty, very dishevelled, but with a victorious gleam in his eye.

'Mum,' he yelled, 'I did it! I fixed my eye on that line and no one was going to drag me down, and I made it!'

We need spiritual determination in fixing our eyes on Jesus, to overcome the people and circumstances who would seek to pull us down. In his early days playing rugby, Duncan would attempt to bring his opponent down by lawful or unlawful tackles. The over-ruling principle was to stop the other man scoring. Satan is our enemy and he is intelligent, devious and diabolical in his endeavours to drag us down and spoil our commitment to Jesus. He has no conscience about the havoc he wreaks in your life. He'll stop at nothing to destroy you. He'll throw everything at you. But take heart. You don't score a century in cricket unless you are bowled at. Every ball bowled has an evil intention. To get you out! But every ball you strike encourages you to carry on. Confidence builds as victory continues to be your experience. But take care,

If you think you are standing firm, be careful that you don't fall
(1 Cor 10:12).

The meaning behind the word 'fix' is to set our gaze
steadfastly upon Jesus. To deliberately look away from
all else that would divert us. 'Fix' is not a fleeting glance,
but a concentrated studied gaze. Our elder son is totally
absorbed by aircraft. His binoculars are never far from
his side. A peaceful afternoon will often be disrupted, as
he hurtles through the patio doors, opening them first,
into the garden and concentrates every eye muscle up
through those binoculars onto the tiny speck moving
towards Hurn Airport. From those few concentrated
seconds he can tell you the registration number, what it
is conveying, where it has come from, and the colour of
the pilot's socks!

With our concentration on the 'Author and Perfecter
of our Faith' we will experience the peace that only God
can give in tough and tiring times.

You will keep in perfect peace him whose mind is steadfast,
because he trusts in you.

Isaiah 26 verse 3 is a picture of a ship's crew warned of
an imminent storm. Everything loose on board is strapped down. This will give it a better chance of coming
through the buffeting undamaged. The storms of life
can, and do, knock the stuffing out of us. Not only
should our eyes be fixed on Jesus but we should secure
ourselves to him. To be trapped in a long queue of
holiday traffic is tiring and ulcer building. Car bumpers
welded together by exhaust fumes, don't exactly inspire
us. Yet far above the poisonous fumes and fraying tempers, the Police Helicopter has a bird's-eye view of the
whole situation. They can identify the cause of the

delays and should be able to unjam the jam! Sadly, the car drivers can see the chopper in the sky but cannot communicate with it. They are therefore robbed of the opportunity of knowing what is happening up ahead. How thrilling to know that we fix our gaze upon a God who has all of our life in view and can communicate with us about it. If our life is seen as a jigsaw puzzle, then God sees all the pieces slotting into place perfectly. Separated from the others, an isolated piece may seem disjointed and ugly, but in relation to the overall picture it fits perfectly! Never forget that God has all the pieces even if you do not have the total picture. He is putting it all together. At times that may actually be a painful process. You may be tempted to ask 'Why does it have to be this way, Lord?' If you do, be prepared not to get satisfactory answers. 'Why' is the difficult question. Jesus cried out

My God, my God, why have you forsaken me? (Mt 27:46)

The answer he received was silence! God is a God of mystery as well as of miracle. Most of us can handle miracles better than we can cope with mysteries. We expect God to roll back the Red Sea and to feed a crowd with a lad's lunch. But we are bewildered by God's silence and apparent inconsistencies in dealing with people (Heb 11:32-38). Fortunately he knows what he is doing, and the things that happen to us are not always for us. They can be for other people through us. Our lives may minister the comfort of Christ to those who suffer, because we have previously known that same comfort in suffering (2 Cor 1:3-5). There are no negative experiences with God. Everything is redeemable. Feeling fit to drop? Then fall into the arms of God's grace.

7

FIT FOR NOTHING

There are special moments in our lives that we love to capture on film. The ecstatic joy of arms flung high in victory after a hard game, family reunions, beautiful sunsets, rough seas pounding the beach, and the first earthly moments of a new baby. Unfortunately I am not very adept at photography. As a result many of my finest hours or minutes are only recorded in my memory.

One particular experience still evokes exhilaration and pleasure each time I recall it. With a large group of young people I had spent an exhausting day climbing up Snowdon in North Wales. As we rounded the final curve on our homeward stretch, we were very hot and weary, with our lips parched by the dust we threw up as we scrambled and slid down the mountain. What a view confronted us! There spread out before us was the most inviting expanse of water. The lake shimmered in the sunshine. None of us could resist the silent invitation offered by that cool, still water. Only boots and jackets were torn off as we plunged into the water. True, we only had a few moments of refreshment and sheer enjoyment but they are moments that live on in my memory!

What a gift our memories are. Without having to flick a switch, or turn the pages of a photograph album, we can speed through the years and in full colour relive our joys and achievements.

Occasionally, though, we are very thankful no one is around to record our failures and disappointments. I'll not forget the day I sat completely shattered and demoralized in the school cloakroom. I had retreated there after a confrontation with my form teacher. She had just knocked me for six! My usual carefree approach to life had gone horribly wrong. She penetratingly analysed my attitude to work, relationships, authority and my future. Her final assessment, spoken more in exasperation than bitterness rang in my ears:

'You are fit for nothing but to play games!'

I knew that last phrase didn't only apply to my sporting activities, but to every other department of my life. Away from the crowds in that basement cloakroom I faced up to myself. I felt totally useless, inadequate and a complete failure. School life droned on above my head as God stopped me in my tracks, and through my misery and sense of rejection he gently brought me to my senses. Although the first fifteen years of my life had been happy, I had generously wasted my time, talent, money, and the patience of all who cared for me. Where was it all leading to? What could God do with so irresponsible a teenager? I couldn't concentrate for more than ten minutes at a stretch and I hated academic work. My passionate love was for sport. In the years since those desolate, empty moments of despair, I have discovered that God never makes a mistake. He created us with gifts, talent and character. I had no blinding Damascus Road revelation in that empty cloakroom. The raincoats and shoe bags hung silently veiling my misery but as I climbed the steps out of that basement, I began to emerge from the mess I was making of my life. In desperation I asked God to take what little I had and use it. Praise God! He's in the life construction business! He delights in taking our inadequacies and making them into his opportunities. He fashions triumphs out of our tears and tragedies. The sensational and spectacular are not what he is looking for, but the simple acts of faith which are so special to him. Ability is not all-important to God. Yet it is not unimportant because he gave us the intelligence we possess, and he expects us to use it for his honour in his world. The vital thing is that we make available to God our abilities, such as they are, and then see his power use and develop them. Never underestimate God's power to use what you have to offer, however small.

David offered God his skill with stones and a sling and Goliath fell dead. Shamgar used his ox-goad and the enemies of Israel were slain. A little boy gave up his packed lunch and saw it miraculously multiplied beyond his wildest dreams to feed 5,000 people. If you feel you are fit for nothing, then you have reached an evaluation of yourself that makes you fit for God's service. He chooses the weak so that all the glory comes to him. As we throw our lot in with God, he gets his loving, creative hands on us to mould and shape us into someone useful and beautiful, fit for him. As the song reminds us:

Something beautiful, something good
All my confusion, He understood.
All I had to offer Him was brokenness and strife
But He made something beautiful of my life.

William and Gloria Gaither © Coronation Music Ltd, 30 Winchester Road, Chawton, Alton, Hants GU34 1RX.

During a trip to the Lake District we joined the long queue of cars making for Kendal. The rain had been heavy and tourists from all directions homed in on the town. They swarmed like bees into the multi-storey car park. Rain is no respecter of early closing days, so with no library open I sat in the back of my car writing. I watched the monotonous procession of cars circling endlessly round the concrete maze searching for parking space. They seemed to be on a giant helter skelter. How often we circle endlessly round trying to find our position in life, growing increasingly tired and frustrated, longing to feel secure and useful. Two verses in the Bible have steered thousands safely into personal security and fulfilment:

> Trust in the Lord with all your heart and lean not on your own understanding; in all your ways acknowledge him and he will make your paths straight (Prov 3:5-6).

However confused and bewildered we might feel, there is a clear path ahead. A path of fulfilment, satisfaction, challenge, and security. Sometimes it will involve us in grief and pain. Always there will be discipline and hard work but the end product is intended to be our spiritual fitness and usefulness to God.

My teacher said that I was only fit to 'play games' but when I gave that flimsy ability to God, he motivated me to study in order to teach others. Three years of anatomy, physiology, psychology and education as well as a wide strenuous physical education programme involved me in such a discipline of mind and body that my character was literally chiselled out and then knocked into shape. Through sport and especially games, I learnt the wider basics of team work and the importance and value of encouraging and appreciating others.

Many of the men and women God used are first seen behind the scenes. Gideon was threshing the corn, hiding away from the Midianites. Ruth was gleaning corn in the fields. Jonah was running away from a divine commission. Samuel was sleeping in the temple. David was alone on the Judean hills caring for the family flock of sheep.

Two apparently insignificant characters are a continual encouragement to me. The poor widow spoken about in Luke 21 verses 2-4 would have certainly passed unnoticed if it hadn't been for the searching compassionate eye of Jesus. As she shuffled past she gave all she possessed in surrendering those two copper coins. Similarly the lady with her precious ointment and tears in Mark 14 verses 3-9 would have been shoved heartlessly aside if it hadn't been for Jesus' words of rebuke to the offenders. 'Leave her alone, why are you bothering her? She has done a beautiful thing to me.' Their simple acts of love magnify the fact that these two women did all they could for, and gave all they had to Jesus. That's all God requires of us. We don't have to strive to be what we are not. Neither do we have to struggle to achieve a fantastic performance beyond our capabilities.

I have discovered that my weaknesses and failures are a far more precious gift to God than my strengths and successes. An important section of my training at college was teaching physically and mentally handicapped children. The months I spent in their company hold some bittersweet memories. I am convinced that as a teacher I learned so much more from their lives than they did from mine. In the term leading up to Christmas, I was helping in the preparation of a special Christmas Party for them. Various decorations were constructed, food was prepared and carols rehearsed. One little seven-year-old girl followed all that took place with interest and longing eyes. She had the most incredible smile and was always willing to help. Tragically, progressive muscular dystrophy had moved silently through her body and left her with only slight finger movements. Although she only had a few months to live, she longed to help at the party. For weeks I had sat in the grounds of the college with her and my piano accordion, practising 'Silent Night, Holy Night'. I squeezed the box and with what little power she had left in her fingers, she pressed the right keys. When the great day arrived, it was that fragile body, enclosed in her beautiful party dress, that stole the show. 'Silent Night' has never been sung like it was that day. Why? Because one little frail life had done what she could and given everything she had in doing it.

The woman with her precious ointment poured out upon Jesus the equivalent of a whole year's wages. Surrender is the qualification needed to be fit for God's use. Not only our abilities and gifts; but our failures and disappointments; the heartaches and bereavements; the glorious configuration of experiences that make us uniquely us. In surrender lies relief and fulfilment.

So why do we hesitate? Why do we continually avoid or ignore the dedicated life? What stops us giving all we have? The answer is sin. That is not a welcome word in our sophisticated society, but it renders the Christian ineffective in service because it breaks his fellowship with God.

American boxer, Harvey Gatler, holds a most unenviable boxing record. The bell got the first round under way. He moved from his corner, circled around, then swung a right hand at his opponent. He missed, slipped, fell and ended up knocking himself out. The referee counted him out. The whole contest lasted 27 seconds! I wonder how he explained it all to his family.

If it was sin that brutally nailed Jesus to a rough cross and rammed needle-sharp thorns into his head, how can he use a life still riddled with and condoning it? We knock ourselves out time and time again by persisting in sinful actions, attitudes and activities. But 'If we confess our sin, he is faithful and just and will forgive us our sins and purify us from all unrighteousness' (1 Jn 1:9). Accumulated and unconfessed sin disqualifies us from useful service. The combination of a drought and a dustman's strike taught us much about the dangers of uncleared rubbish. Newspapers in their ones and twos presented no problem yet as they piled up so did the dilemma. So too the minor irritations of life. The niggling jealousies, the little white lies and the few harsh words all appear to be nothing to worry about at first. But if they are left they will multiply, crowd out love and forgiveness and cause endless hurt.

In one of our previous houses, our water was heated by a large old-fashioned kitchen boiler. One morning Doug cleared the ashes out from beneath the boiler and carried them out to our already overflowing dustbin. Juggling with the full tray and the lid of the dustbin is never easy. It is almost impossible. The first warning I got that my husband was in trouble was a strangulated cry. Then, covered from head to toe in white ash, he appeared at the back door. My gales of laughter did not bless him. Nothing short of a bath and a complete change of clothes could free him from that clinging ash. The coal that had been so useful bringing warmth and comfort was now nothing but an annoying, suffocating dust. So much that is useful in us is spoilt by our pride, wrong attitudes, and moaning. These destroying sins, if not dealt with, infiltrate every part of our lives and smother our spiritual service.

Bottles and cans posed the next problem. We smashed, crushed, and hammered them flat. Still they mounted up. Empty, useless containers! So much that is empty and useless can occupy our lives. Stamping on them and crushing them with human resolve and determination will not adequately remove them from our lives. They have to be spiritually overcome.

With mounting temperatures, came increased anxiety over rotting food. Suddenly, what before had been classed as 'little leftovers' became a big health hazard. The Song of Solomon reminds us that 'little foxes spoil the vines' (2:15), and Ecclesiastes states that 'dead flies cause the ointment of the apothecary to send forth a stinking savour' (Eccles 10:1 AV). Not dead elephants or giraffes, but tiny flies. The flies got trapped as they landed upon the ointment setting in the jar. Trapped, they died in it and caused it to lose its pleasant aroma. It's the little sins that cause a spiritual health hazard in our lives. The insensitive remarks, the carelessness about our devotional life, thoughtlessness in relationships, laziness, unkindness towards our parents and a critical spirit.

Only when the dustmen returned to work and removed the rubbish which had piled up were we free from the mess. But the clean up at the end of the strike had to be supported by the regular weekly disposal of waste. On the cross, Jesus the Saviour dealt with sin and now gives to those who receive him and believe on his name, the right to be called sons of God (Jn 1:12).

Joined to God by the chain of salvation, we maintain that relationship through the thread of fellowship. 1 Samuel 2:8 says 'He raises the poor from the dust and lifts the needy from the ash heap'. The daily forsaking of sin is vital to a healthy friendship with God.

Mounting the rostrum at the Olympic Games to receive a gold medal must be the supreme moment in any athlete's career. The ultimate reward. As their national flag is raised and the national anthem echoes round the stadium their hearts deserve to swell with pride. Which of us has not dreamed of such a moment?

It is natural for self to seek the prominent place. At the centre of sIn is I. Until Christ occupies the dominant position we will never give all we have to God. Continual discipline is needed to keep Christ central in our life. Each time our will crosses with God's will and we choose God's will, we have learned, in that moment, to die to self.

Nevertheless, we do have another foe, Satan. About him, C. S. Lewis has rightly said, we make two major mistakes. One is to pay no attention to him, to deny his existence. The other is to give too much attention to him, to overstate the case for him. Jesus never took him for granted. He recognized his power and authority but overcame it. So can we through the word and by the Spirit (Mt 4:1). Because the One who is in us is greater than he who is in the world, victory comes as we yield to him who is within us.

8

FIT FOR A KING

There was an air of anticipation and excitement about those seven fourteen-year-olds on that blustery March morning. This was the day we had worked and trained so hard for. Those early morning starts, the circuit training, step-ups and stamina building were all behind us now.

Our netball team travelled to the host school, where the Surrey County Netball Tournament was to be held. This annual event was an important date on the sports calendar of the schools in South London and Surrey. We were fully aware of the honour that was ours to represent our school. We had approached the first rounds in fear and trepidation. Now the underdogs had made it all the way to the finals. Today it was all or nothing. We were determined to win!

Our confidence grew as we made our way successfully through the early rounds and we were in sight of the semi-finals. In our bright red gym shirts and royal blue games skirts we were now seen as a possible threat to the usual winners of the tournament. It was rare for an unknown team to reach the finals. Thus with jangling nerves, we took our place in the final. All the participating schools crowded round that court. The tournament holders were our opponents and appeared to be twice our size. Throwing caution to the wind, we gave that match everything we'd got. The score see-sawed and reflected the closeness of the match. With the scores level, just a few seconds remaining, our shooter paused to aim. The silence was electrifying. Tired players held their breath, and you could almost hear their hearts pounding inside their rib cages. My eyes were closed and I couldn't bear to watch. I listened: the swish of the net, the cheers and the final whistle told me all I wanted to know. We had won!

There was a great celebration as we returned to our school. We were summoned to the gymnasium. Through the door strode our games teacher. The two single words she uttered, 'Well done,' meant more to us than the trophy itself. We had done it all for her and in our little lives she was number one! She had taught us all we knew about the game of netball. She had exercised endless patience and understanding in developing our skills. As Squash Champion of the United Kingdom, she knew about total dedication and taught it to us. She had a tremendous impact on my life.

Young people are natural disciples. They seek a cause to commit themselves to. A person to follow. An objective to achieve. Sport and pop stars dictate tastes in music, fashion and behaviour. Thousands follow their example. We all long to extract the most from life and search everywhere for something or someone who has the secret of life satisfaction. In the world of fitness and skill, we look to Jane Fonda, Martina Navratilova, Chris Lloyd, Sebastian Coe or Daly Thompson. The scientific and academic worlds present us with the example of Albert Einstein, Michael Faraday and Blaise Pascal. The social climbers can be read about in the gossip columns and magazines. The spiritual giants, such as Amy Carmichael, Mary Slessor, Jim Elliot, Billy

Graham and Luis Palau are tremendous examples and a challenge to all of us. But there is only one man who ever lived that can demand and deserve our worship. Only one man who can enable us to live life as it was intended to be lived. He said, 'I have come that they may have life, and have it to the full' (Jn 10:10). He wasn't speaking to graves, but to living beings. So the life he is talking about is something more than physical life. It is eternal life and that does not mean quantity but quality. With Jesus at the centre of our lives we are fit for the King, we have worth and value before God. He sees us as fit for his service. In Luke 2:52 we have a picture of someone who has all round fitness:

Jesus grew in all wisdom (academic fitness) and stature (physical fitness), and in favour with God (spiritual fitness) and man (social fitness).

If all that Jesus claims is true, his life deserves closer scrutiny. What is it that makes his life unique and different from all other lives?

First, Jesus was *God willing to become man.* Although I have known this fact for many years, it is more incredible to me now than on that first Christmas when it was explained to me. Could that tiny baby actually be God himself? The Creator willing to be created. The King willing to be a subject. The greatest willing to be the smallest. The strongest willing to be the weakest. The richest willing to be the poorest. And above all, the sinless willing to become sin. But why?

Let two small, painful illustrations from our family life help with the answer. They are about tadpoles and baby birds! Stephen had closely observed the intriguing development of those tiny creatures in the fish bowl. Excitement had greeted the appearance of tails and legs.

But one morning there was a strange silence. I investigated and discovered some of the tadpoles crazily swimming around in the bowl. The remainder lay on the bottom, legless. A young lad's enquiring mind had decided to see if new legs would grow. He had innocently killed them in the process.

The second incident involved Duncan. As a family we had watched a bird build a nest in our small apple tree. We carefully kept our distance when she laid her eggs. Duncan watched from his bedroom window. He saw the tiny birds emerge and the regular feeding of those fragile balls of feathers. Early one morning his curiosity proved too great for him. Scaling the tree, he planted two fat juicy worms into the fledglings' welcoming beaks. The mother fled, resulting in the death of the little birds. It was a heart-breaking lesson to learn. I tried, very inadequately, to explain to the boys the reason for those deaths and their part in it. But what about the tadpoles and the mother bird? Ridiculously I longed to be able to communicate with them also. To enter their world of confusion and pain and say sorry and try to put things right.

But even if I could have become a bird or a tadpole, I still would not have had the answer to their dilemma. Sin wreaks havoc in human experience, creating chaos, pain and confusion, separating man from his Maker. God alone could conceive the solution to this dilemma. He took upon himself a body like ours. He became one of us! He entered our experience by way of natural birth. He had his nappies changed. He cut teeth, learned to talk and walk. He had his face washed and his nose wiped. He experienced the rough and tumble of family life. He learned a trade working with his carpenter father. He matured into manhood, with the accompanying responsibility. An extraordinary life—because it was a life lived as God intended, without sin. The only life lived with its death in view. A death for others (1 Cor 15:3). A death that brought eternal benefit to others (Rom 6:23).

Second, Jesus was a man *willing to be behind the scenes*. In total contrast to other biographies there is very little biblical detail concerning his early life. His birth is briefly and swiftly covered. Virtually all of his teen and twenty years are passed over in silence. The focus of interest is upon the last three years of his life. Those years behind the scenes were formative ones. He fasted, prayed and was tested and toughened. He lived in submission to his earthly parents. He experienced human weariness and pain. He grew physically. He was involved with people, living with them. He got stuck into our life. But we must not forget, that although he was behind the scenes, he was always in control of the situation. He was moving all the scenes he was behind. His goal was the cross and the defeat of Satan and sin.

Thirdly, Jesus was a man *willing to break the silence*!

For two years after I asked Jesus to come into my life, I remained silent about that commitment. I was like an Arctic river, frozen at the mouth! I grew up in a Christian family, and by human standards I had no tremendous conversion. I expressed no overwhelming joy and saw no blinding flashes of lightning. I heard no voices. But I look back on that quiet transaction between me and God with some satisfaction now. I didn't understand it then, nor did I want to talk about it. I was silent, hesitant, and apologetic. As God continued his silent work in me, there came a time when I was forced to break that silence. It happened at the end of a hockey match, and drew from my friend an embarrassed retort that left me standing strangely at peace. I knew that at last I had done what God expected me to do. I learned that God never calls us to something without providing us with the power to do it. At the right moment Jesus emerged from anonymity to be baptized by the controversial John the Baptist before hundreds of people. This authority summoned a strong-willed fisherman like Peter to follow him. Without hesitation and with patient resolution he answered the critical questions of the Pharisees. Jesus broke the silence with actions that spoke louder than words. Sadly most of the world was deaf.

It is said that in one of his early performances, the late Richard Burton scrubbed the floor in such a way that he 'had the audience riveted!' Wherever Jesus appeared, his life and teaching demanded attention and response.

Fourthly, Jesus was a man *willing to be a servant*. Christ gave himself to others in his life and for others in his death. He was a servant at the beck and call of everyone. 'Everyone is looking for you' (Mk 1:37). A crowd came to him (Mk 2:13). People came to him from everywhere (Mk 3:8). A large crowd followed him (Mk 3:7). Those who were ill kept pushing their way to him in order to touch him (Mk 3:10). Such a large crowd, no time to eat (Mk 3:20). He taught his disciples how to be servants (Jn 13). He took a towel and washed their feet. The Creator served the created. As Christians, we tend to believe in the principle of servanthood until we are asked to act like servants.

Fifthly, Jesus was a man *willing to die for our sin*. He didn't have to die! He was without sin and 'the wages of sin is death' (Rom 3:23).

The death he died was for us sinful human beings. It took him through the mockery of a trial. The merciless scourging. The excruciating pain of the cross. The spiritual agony of bearing our sin. He suffered physically, mentally, socially, and spiritually. But he could still say,

Father, forgive them, for they do not know what they are doing (Lk 23:34).

He alone was fit enough to make that sacrifice. His blood alone can cleanse us from sin and bring peace to our conscience. Simple words summarize it all:

There was no other good enough
To pay the price of sin,
He only could unlock the gate
Of heaven and let us in.

As we watch top musicians, sportsmen, and star performers of any kind, we begin to feel totally inadequate, because our endeavours and achievements seem pathetic by comparison, and too easily we lose heart and give up. Looking at the example of Jesus might well induce despair in us. It wouldn't surprise me to hear some say 'I couldn't live up to such a standard' or 'I'm not perfect like he was.'

We don't have to lose heart, because finally, Jesus was a man *willing to bring his solution* to all our inadequacies. Jesus said,

No one who puts his hand to the plough and looks back is fit for service in the kingdom of God (Lk 9:62).

From the moment he was born, Jesus' life was set like a furrow. He fixed his eyes on the cross. He ploughed straight through death and out the other side. He didn't look back—*he came back*.

After the resurrection Jesus ascended into heaven. He sent his Spirit to fill his people so that he could continue his work through them. The ministry he started in the flesh, he now continues in us by his Spirit.

High diving is a very spectacular sport. The combination of poise, co-ordination and timing all contribute to a breathtaking spectacle. Shortly after watching a world-class high diving competition, I visited a pool with a ten metre high diving board. With the memory of those incredible dives clearly etched in my mind, I started to climb up the ladder to the board high above my head. How I longed to dive just like those world-class divers. Deep down I knew this was impossible. But what if by some miracle one of those divers could have lived inside my body. All their wealth of training and ability would become mine. Their eyes could judge the height through mine. Their disciplined concentration could harness my lack of application. Their agility and dexterity could engineer the dive. I could have performed a perfect armstand, double somersault with pyke! I might have even managed a back one and a half somersault with two and a half twists! It's amazing what the imagination can do for you! The brutal reality is that as soon as I stepped onto that ten metre board, I was almost paralysed with fright by the height. It was impossible for me to jump let alone dive. I also had another problem. I couldn't turn around and descend the ladder. It took all my self control to return to the ground literally shaking like a leaf.

In contrast, we are not in the world of fantasy, but living in the world of glorious fact when we discover that God can live in us, through the power of the Holy Spirit. Not to help us perform incredible dives without discipline and training, but to enable us to reach our full potential in day-to-day living. We can't survive the pain of bereavement, but he can through us. We can't cope with continual destructive criticism, but he can through us. We can't heal a marriage relationship, face failure in exams, kick drink or drugs, we can't write a book, but he can through us.

All the limitless power, wisdom and patience of one all-seeing, all-knowing God is put at our disposal when we allow the Holy Spirit to live his life through us.

Because I appreciate wood, I have been given bowls, shelves, trays, tables, spoons and even spectacle frames! But never a staircase! Until we moved into our present home. There it was, a beautiful pine staircase. The grain and knots were beautiful. I longed to see them enhanced by the polish. I swallowed my disappointment when the workmen stained it a hideous red by mistake! Removing that stain would be almost impossible, I was told.

Then J.R. appeared on the scene. Equipped with time, patience, and a determination I have rarely seen, our good carpenter friend placed a huge contraption on the floor, along with dust sheets and sandpaper. The heavy, cumbersome piece of machinery turned out to be an industrial orbital sander and apparently was the answer to my problem. I was eager to help with the marathon task. So I picked up a sheet of sandpaper. Gritting my teeth, I set to work. Twenty long minutes and ten sore fingers later I surveyed a tiny patch of red streaked wood. It looked worse than the original effort and I could have wept with frustration. Out of curiosity I picked up the sander. Noticing a sanding pad in place, I reckoned that with the extra weight the job would be made easier. I ignored the flex and plug—that was for the expert! It didn't take long for me to realize that the extra weight was on my arms not on the wood! Exhausted, I gave up until with infinite patience J.R. explained to me that the industrial sander was never invented to be operated manually. That heavy awkward equipment became surprisingly light and extremely effective when operated by the greater power of electricity.

Spiritually we can't operate manually either. Our

feeble efforts are doomed to failure and leave us spiritually sore. There is a greater power available to us. For years I ignored the ministry of the Holy Spirit, through lack of understanding and fear. I didn't have to fully comprehend the working of the orbital sander nor be an expert in the science of electricity to see the amazing job they did when united. Until I meet Jesus face to face, I will never fathom the full and free life he has given me nor understand the power and indwelling presence of the Holy Spirit, but lack of knowledge doesn't prevent me experiencing that power flooding through me. When I am united to Christ he works through me and I discover that I am not fit for nothing! I am fit for the King.

9

FIT AND REFRESHED

The heat was bouncing off the tarmac in Los Angeles, as the lady marathon runners neared the end of their most gruelling Olympic ordeal. Instead of the rousing cheers that greeted the other runners as they entered the stadium, a sympathetic silence welcomed Gaby Anderson-Schiess, the Swiss runner. Her exhausted, unco-ordinated movements drew an agonized sigh of relief from the capacity crowd, as she completed the distance and collapsed into the arms of the anxious medical team. Throughout the long, draining miles, water had been consumed by and sponged and splashed over the runners. But Gaby's condition accentuated the importance of the correct water balance in the human body system. The body is seventy-five per cent water and the blood is a colossal ninety per cent water. A diminished body fluid reduces the capacity of the performance. Within hours of medical attention, Gaby was interviewed on television. Her appearance and reactions were quite normal, and although she had received medical treatment, including rest, the main reason for her remarkable recovery was H_2O.

Water is an essential part of our diet. It refreshes,

strengthens, revitalizes and cleans the system. Any lack of it is soon apparent.

Our green and pleasant England rarely experiences serious water shortage. But it was during a notably dry spell that our family went on holiday to the normally rain drenched Lake District. We were staying in a picturesque spot just above Dove Cottage in Grasmere, the birthplace of the poet William Wordsworth. It had been a long hot summer with temperatures soaring into the 80s. Daily we plotted our walks over the fells with waterfalls and tarns in mind. The clear weather enabled us to appreciate the beauty of the rugged fells. How thankfully we plunged into the welcoming lakes. Fatigue, thirst, aches and pains were all forgotten as the clear, cool water covered us. Towards the end of our holiday, we planned a longer walk over a new route. Setting off early, the day stretched before us shimmering with promised heat. Our rucksacks were bulging with flasks of tea and bottles of lemonade. The map promised several streams and waterfalls amongst the fells before our first tarn. Our spirits were high as we scrambled up the first incline. The scars of the long drought were more evident on this climb with cracks and dust everywhere. Springs and streams were reduced to trickles of water or just dry beds. As the sun mounted high in the sky so the level of our personal drink supply lowered, until the last drop trickled down our throats. The natural exuberance of our boys was silenced as they panted their way up and down hill. With each fell we mounted and each bend we rounded hopes sank as no lake or stream materialized. As we sank exhausted into the coarse dry turf, sucking our last apples, we scanned the haze ahead for other walkers. Nothing. No figures, no distant voices. We were lost, tired, and very, very thirsty! Anyone viewing us would have seen a defeated, dejected family swallowed up by a dry and dusty landscape.

Recalling that scene years later reminds me of the desperate spiritual thirst experienced by groups across Great Britain today. Our comparatively tiny, water surrounded island experiences a dryness that causes spiritual dehydration. Family groups, social groups, political groups, pop groups and tragically some church groups cry out for a deeper, more satisfying experience of life. Their thirst is not quenched by power, riches, fame, sex, knowledge, violence or religion. The cracks in our parched land are seen in the rising divorce figures, the deep rooted racial prejudice, the frightening child abuse and the decline in verbal and ethical values. The population is left panting and longing for peace, purpose and real life.

Water is the most important element in the world. A seed cannot sprout, a foetus cannot grow, and human beings cannot exist without it. Life depends upon it. Without it we die. Spiritually, we depend on Living Water! Palestine was a very dry country. Rainwater was collected in cisterns. The people were constantly searching for the living springs. As a result, water in the Old Testament became a picture and symbol of God, the giver and sustainer of life. Speaking of God, the psalmist says, 'you let us drink from the river of your goodness. You are the source of all life' (Ps 36:8-9 GNB). Isaiah gives thanks to God and says, 'As fresh water brings joy to the thirsty, so God's people rejoice when he saves them' (Is 12:3 GNB). How can we get the help we need? Let's go back to our experience in the Lake District.

Three factors saved the day for us. First the map. In desperation we spread it out on the ground and studied it carefully. Because we had failed to consult the map regularly, we had wandered away from the right path.

After some discussion we set off on a corrected route, in a revised direction. This time we had the map folded to the right section, and always to hand. After walking for about half an hour, our boys were wilting visibly. Doug tried to encourage them, as he constantly looked at the map,

'Just one more little climb, lads. Over that hill is the Lake!' Duncan collapsed in a heap muttering,

'I don't believe you!'

I was inclined to agree with him but wisely kept quiet. Here was no place for a family argument. Now the second factor appeared, a dog. Over the hill he raced, closely followed by his owner. No ordinary hound this. He was the most beautiful creature I had ever seen—not because he was a pedigree German Shepherd or a Yorkshire Terrier, but because he was saturated from nose to tail with water! He stopped by us, shook his gleaming coat and sent sprays of water everywhere. As the Barnett family accelerated up the hill, the dog's owner greeted us with a short welcome sentence,

'Not far now!'

He too was soaked. Water ran down his face from his drenched hair. Duncan was first over the hill, his unbelief disappearing as fast as his clothes, as he fell into the lake.

The third factor now comes into operation. What we saw on the map and in the soaking twosome, what we heard from Doug and the owner of the dog, we had to act upon. In no time at all we had all plunged into the lake and drunk from an ice cold spring. God provides us with a map for life's journey. Careful study and consultation of the Bible shows that the Old Testament points forward to Jesus, showing him to be the fulfilment of the promises of God to bring water to a thirsty land and life to a dying people. Jesus said,

I am the way and the truth and the life. No-one comes to the Father except through me (Jn 14:6).

Two thousand years before our walk in the lakeland hills, Jesus had walked from Judaea to Galilee. He knew tiredness and thirst in a much hotter climate than ours. In the fierce heat of noon, he rested by a well at Sychar and asked a Samaritan woman for a drink. She questioned him and Jesus said,

If only you knew what God gives and who it is that is asking you for a drink, you would ask him, and he would give you life-giving water (Jn 4:10 GNB).

Jesus called himself many things to help us understand his character. He said 'I am the light of the world' (Jn 8:12) and 'I am the bread of life' (Jn 6:35). But he never said 'I am the living water.' He informs us that he has the living water to give to us.

Whoever is thirsty should come to me and drink. As the scripture says. 'Whoever believes in me, streams of life-giving water will pour out from his heart.' Jesus said this about the Spirit, which those who believed in him were going to receive. At that time the Spirit had not yet been given, because Jesus had not been raised to glory (Jn 7:37-39 GNB).

After years of spiritual drought, I believe there is a rain cloud on the horizon. As all kinds and classes of people open up the Bible again and begin to discuss the person of Jesus and discover his love and salvation, and as they drink deeply of that spiritual life-giving water, they become living proof that God is still at work in this world. That lone man with his dog didn't have to try to convince us that there was water ahead. Neither did he have to push us up and over the hill! One look at his soaking body did the trick. The water spoke for itself! In the same way we must let the Holy Spirit speak and work for himself. We underestimate the power God has given to us at conversion. We crowd him out with our fleshly efforts. Just as God waits patiently for us to invite him into our lives, so he continues to wait for us to ask him to fill and overflow us with his Holy Spirit. God promises,

> I will give water to the thirsty land and make streams flow on the dry ground. I will pour out my power on your children and my blessing on your descendants. They will thrive like well-watered grass, like willows by the streams of running water. (Is 44:3-4 GNB).

Do the people around us find a path to God because of us? Is the impact of the Holy Spirit obvious in our living? Do our neighbours and family get introduced to Jesus by us? As the Holy Spirit fills and affects every part of our lives, we will become channels of living water for others.

We left that lake fully refreshed and were able to encourage many other parched walkers and point them in the direction of refreshment. It wasn't long though, before the scorching sun, and the steady exercise of walking had dried us out and we were looking for our next swim. Life has a habit of drying us out physically and mentally. If we are not continually asking God to fill us on a daily basis, we will resort to our own strength. With the result that we quickly grow very weary. It is not a once-for-all experience. We need constant filling or we will dry up! Paul urges the Ephesians to 'be being filled with the Spirit' (Eph 5:18). It is a continuous command! We cannot depend upon special events for our spiritual highs! Spring Harvest, the Dales, the Downs, Filey, Greenbelt, Keswick, this convention, that conference,

Holiday Centres and Royal Week can all become special Lakes in the Spiritual District. All these events will build us up and refresh us but the deep work is the continuous walking in the Spirit. Without the latter we become rocking-horse Christians. We get on the horse, have a lot of fun, expend a great deal of energy moving it up and down and make a lot of noise as we ride the horse. When we dismount, we discover that we haven't been anywhere, we are still in the same place as when we started! It's of little help to us to move in all the best evangelical circles, if we don't move forward. 'Grow in grace' (2 Pet 3:18) is the word we need to heed.

The days of bedtime stories have long since passed for our boys but it always amazed me to discover their favourites. A peaceful night's rest would only come after battles, knights in armour, and hair-raising adventures. They would turn over with a contented sigh and sink into a deep, untroubled sleep. I would return to a lonely vigil by the fire imagining all manner of shapes within the flames! I remember reading time after time about a siege. The advancing army would surround the castle. The occupants of the castle had closed all possible entrances. The drawbridge was raised and all was ominously silent as night descended. The invaders simply dammed up any streams or rivers flowing into the defended area. Then they could just sit and wait for the defenders to surrender. Victory depended on the latter's water supply. To be totally dependent upon outside water resources meant surrender came very quickly. However, the defenders would have been able to resist for a much longer period if they had had a deep well of water in the castle. They would have been a force to be reckoned with whilst they were drawing on that inner source of life and energy. If we depend on outward circumstances and events to supply our spiritual energy we will become spiritual yo-yos, growing increasingly discontented. We must draw daily from the deep well placed within us, allowing the Holy Spirit to saturate us with his wisdom, refreshment, encouragement and power, making us fit and keeping us refreshed at all times and in all circumstances.

10

FIT FOR THE FAMILY

It had started peacefully, that game of cards. Four children playing together on the lounge floor. I was alerted to the impending storm by the raised voices.

'You give that card back to me. It's mine!'

'No it's not! I had it first!'

'You're a cheat!'

'Don't you dare call me a cheat!'

'Cheat, cheat, cheat!'

With that, World War Three commenced. As the furniture got rearranged and tempers rose, I donned my supergirl suit and intervened. Separating the contestants and keeping them from each other's throats, I posed an innocent adult question. 'What game are you children playing that causes such aggravation and hostility?' The oldest girl looked at me with unbelief on her face. She pushed her crumpled cards into my hand and stormed out, calling for her mum. The others processed after her. I paused and then considered the cards. The plastic smile of childhood greeted me. Memories flooded back of the hours I'd spent playing the same game. The name of the game? Happy Families!

Sadly the family unit is far from happy at times. Fighting starts early, rifts soon appear and relationships fold up. Marriage and family life are not games to be played. They are deep, lifetime commitments. Good relationships don't happen automatically. They must be worked at. They take a lifetime to develop. In our disposable society, we make the mistake of easily discarding our commitments and responsibilities along with our rubbish! Strange that we demand high qualifications, years of training, and university degrees for our most responsible jobs and yet no qualifications are required to enter the most demanding of all occupations—marriage and parenthood.

However, the church is beginning to concentrate its energies in this important area. Family life and marriage seminars and teaching weekends are organized where training in family counselling is provided. There is a proliferation of books written from the biological, psychological and religious standpoints. This is an advance I support. But when the crunch comes, our fitness for marriage and family life is closely related to our relationship with God. He is a God of relationships, who is actively involved with his universe, and the people he created.

He brought Eve to Adam because he was concerned that Adam had no suitable friend and companion amongst the animals. He created a team who could love and enjoy each other's company. But it was a God-dependent relationship. He was central to it. Tragically Adam and Eve became self-centred and then trouble, in the form of sin and all its ramifications, began for the human family. The image of God in man became marred and blurred. God's life and truth was no longer central in man's experience. Man died spiritually. Nevertheless, God did not abandon his creation. If he had started afresh he could not have created a more perfect being! What is better than perfect? A second, a last Adam, enters the world, Jesus. By his life, death and resurrection he offers us his resurrection life in exchange for our spiritual deadness. As we receive Christ, he lives out his life through us. We are united to God, possess life and are daily renewed in the image of our Creator (Col 3). This relationship begins with our response to divine love. From that foundation, our commitment deepens and grows as we learn what it means to become spiritually mature (Col 1).

Love in marriage and family life has got to be more than romantic love. Indeed it's more like an act of the will at times. An act of will that outlives the romantic, emotional feelings, carrying us through the rough times. 'Being in love' is not a sufficient basis for keeping a marriage going. 'Staying in love' is what counts. That brings marriage and family life out of the clouds and sets it squarely on earth. Marriages may well be made in heaven, but they have to operate on earth. Marriage is a high risk business and as such needs the wisdom, insight and instruction of the God who invented it. It has been called 'a complete upheaval in the settled routine of two individuals'. This upheaval can and does have tremendous repercussions, especially when we take on an unrealistic view of that overworked word 'love'. The Beatles told us 'all you need is love'. Experience suggests they were right. Men have fought wars and duels because of it. Women have died for it. Songwriters and poets extol it and despair over it. Children crave it. Teenagers search for it.

In between our emerging birth cries and our final death moans, we seek to experience and express love. Unreserved giving is the true nature of genuine love. Commitment without limitation. There is no substitute for the fulfilment of steady self-giving love returned and rewarded. As I floated up the aisle and into marriage I was neither prepared nor fit for the nineteen years of family life that has followed. Our earthly conception is followed by nine months of preparation before we struggle out into the big world. Before we descend on an unsuspecting school, we have some years of practice in the arts of walking, talking, eating and that never to be forgotten joy of 'potty training'! Preceding our chosen career we enter into years of training. Yet for marriage and family life we so often are flung in at the deep end and it's 'sink or swim!' All we know is what we've been able to cobble together by observation in our own family, by information gleaned from talking to others and discussion of latest theories about marriage love and family life. Does love last? Can it last? Does it really work? Through many personal mistakes and struggles, I have accumulated my own set of 'Love is' cartoons, which I am continually adding to. So far I have discovered that:

Love is: adjusting not agitating. Marriage is a merger of two different people from different family backgrounds, upbringings, standards, values and tastes. Such diverse experience is not easily or quickly welded into one unit. It means tremendous adjustments. Regular reappraisals of our relationship are needed during our lifetime because we are always growing, changing and hopefully maturing. We encounter emotional highs and lows. There are opposite views about important issues. Imagine two hedgehogs caught in a severe snowstorm. How can they survive? Only by huddling close together for warmth. But because they are hedgehogs that needs care and considerable adjustment of their spines to prevent them inflicting pain on the other partner. Marriage has its prickly times when our hackles are up, and we inflict pain upon each other. One route through these times is to try and see things through our partner's eyes. Their opinions, ideas, values and standards may not necessarily be wrong, just different. Pooling our resources in terms of experience and the way we have been taught to approach problems can help enormously.

Growing up in a large active family, we had our fair share of accidents. My mother was a nurse and consequently was used to coping calmly with all kinds of accidents, injuries, bumps and bruises. She never seemed to panic no matter how serious the issue appeared. One day I tumbled head over heels from the top of our stairs to the bottom. Mum greeted me with gales of laughter. It turned my tears of exasperation into laughter in no time at all. The only damage was to my pride. There were times, as children, when we longed for more fuss to be made over our little crises. But we grew up to discover that underneath our Mum's cheerful, lighthearted approach beat a heart of deep, serious concern. She knew that making a big fuss often clouded the incident and prevented proper action being taken swiftly. Growing up with this approach to family incidents, I automatically adopted this 'no fuss' technique. How soon I was to be made aware, by marriage, that this is only one approach. No man, having hammered his nail squarely on the thumb, who goes on an informal and agitated walk around the garden, likes a woman to roar with laughter over it! Least of all my husband, Doug. That wasn't how he had been raised. Of course, I was concerned about his hand but my upbringing sought to diffuse tension and pain with laughter. Doug didn't understand that. It took time and discussion about our upbringing to appreciate why we reacted in such different ways. Learning from each other, we can now harmonize our response to the crises that occur in the lives of our sons. There doesn't have to be conflict when love is adjusting not agitating.

Love is: completing not competing. God designed opposite sexes to complement each other. Joined in marriage we complete each other. Our differences complement and blend two unique individuals into one. But there can also be incompatibilities that divide and cause destructive competition. There was tremendous competition in the early years of our marriage between my relaxed untidiness and Doug's disciplined everything in its place approach. I tried to justify my irresponsibility until I realized my outward expression only declared an inward attitude. We needed to learn from each other. Very slowly I began to practise an inward and outward tidiness and discipline. The competition became an education. As we learned from each other, Doug adopted a more relaxed approach to his rigid routine. It is fascinating to see the different approaches emerging in our boys. We enjoy the times we are able to discuss them as a family. This can only happen when love is completing not competing.

Love is: changing me not changing them! A prayer I utter frequently is 'Lord change me! Make me into the wife my husband needs and the mum my sons need, to become the people you want them to be.' The danger in family relationships is to mould and/or manipulate. 'If only he would. . .' and 'Why can't she. . .?' are familiar cries. True love concerns itself with the enrichment of the one it loves. It doesn't ask what can they do for my benefit but what can I do for them. It is other-centred not self-centred. Love is changing me not changing them!

Jesus, you are changing me.
By your Spirit you're making me like you.

Jesus, you're transforming me,
That your loveliness may be seen in all I do.
You are the potter and I am the clay,
Help me to be willing to let you have your way.
Jesus, you are changing me,
As I let you reign supreme within my heart.

Marilyn Baker © 1981, Coronation Music Ltd, 30 Winchester Road,
Chawton, Alton, Hants GU34 1RX.

Love is: your priority not your property. Possessive-
ness can suffocate and stifle any loving relationship and
in the closeness of family life such love will disrupt and
frustrate. Possessing is part of loving but not as a selfish,
greedy, constricting thing. To understand such an
unselfish togetherness, we have to look at God's love for
us. With his tremendous power he had every right to
possess his creation. He could have made us robots and
ruled us with a computer-like power. Instead he made us
persons, complete with free will and set us loose in his
beautiful world. He took a calculated risk with us. His is
a love that 'lets us go' in order to possess us more fully. If
nineteen years ago Doug had put his foot down, and
commanded 'You will be my wife!', our love would have
been incomplete. I needed to freely respond to his invitation of marriage. That mutual response has to be a
continual one throughout married life. It must flow from
loving freedom and security, not force or confinement.
With our love for God the priority, our ability to love
our families selflessly will be so much greater. As parents, the most difficult exercise in family fitness is to let
our children go. Love encourages them in the plan that
God has for them and doesn't cling selfishly to them.
They are gifts from God and we realize that love is our
priority not our property.

Love is: speaking up not bottling up. The gas boiler is
an important part of our kitchen furniture. It heats our

water and runs the central heating system. To ensure an efficient performance we have a three star service agreement which involves a regular service and check up. Parts are removed and examined carefully. All the clogging fluff and dust that mars the smooth running of the boiler is removed. Weaknesses are pinpointed and dealt with. Kitchen debris is removed. Marriage needs good servicing and careful attention must be given to our communication. Only God can read minds, so we need to share with each other our hopes, fears, and those things that upset and annoy us. Mutual examination of our weaknesses and failures is vital so that the job of cleaning out any festering misunderstandings can take place. Listening is an important element in communication. That means patiently laying aside what we want to say in order to concentrate more fully on what our partner or children are saying to us. Listening enables us to spot that hidden anxiety or fear that cannot be verbalized yet underlies all that is spoken. Keep lines of communication open. Don't encourage the bottling up of hurts, misunderstandings and grievances. That can cause breakdowns in physical and mental health as well as marriage.

After eating large quantities of fresh grass, gas accumulates in the stomach of cows and sheep and will cause their stomachs to balloon up. If the stomach is not pierced in the right place and the gas released, death will follow. That gas is evil smelling and can be ignited! Don't allow festering hurt, bad feelings, misunderstandings and criticism to accumulate in the stomach of family life. Release the pressure. Pierce the affected area with the love of God and wise counsel of your pastor, elders and friends. Talk things out. Pray them through. Get it off your chest—or stomach as the case may be! It will help you keep balance and proportion on the issues. In such a release of hurt, be ready to hear some unpleasant things and avoid igniting over them. Having released and confessed where necessary, rebuild each other! In listening and learning we see that love is speaking up and not bottling up.

Love is: building up and not running down. Encouragement uplifts us especially when it comes from our nearest and dearest. As humans we need constant reassurance. Often those who appear outwardly most confident and well adjusted need lots of supportive encouragement and suffer hardest from destructive criticism. Teenagers tend to draw from their parents negative attitudes and phrases. 'Turn that music down.' 'Why do you mix with those boys! You know I don't like them.' 'Look at the state of your room.' Try being positive for a change. You can always say, 'My, how tidy you've kept the ceiling in your room!' There is always something we can commend if we stop and think about it. There are numerous other ways of building each other up. A bunch of flowers as a love offering not a peace offering; a box of brazil nuts; a day spent fishing; a trip to the airport; a favourite meal; a cup of tea; a smile; a pat on the back will always dislodge a chip on the shoulder; a hug; a single red rose; a listening ear and continuous prayer. Love is building up, not running down.

Love is: accepting not rejecting. 'For better or for worse' seems to echo emptily through countless shattered marriages, broken families and messed up lives. Love is acceptance. In acceptance lies peace. I am learning that lesson, slowly, from my three strongwilled men. Love can so often appear conditional. I will love you: if you have your hair cut; if you speak properly; if you wear my approved clothes; if you pass your exams; if you become a Christian. In correcting our children let's take care to show them that we love them all the time. If your child storms out of the house and slams the door behind him, make sure it's open for his return. Don't lock your child out of your life. Love makes certain there is always a way back. Love doesn't drive people into no hope, no exit situations. God makes it very clear that he hates sin, but he also underscores the fact that he loves us. Practise saying 'I love you' in word and action!! Love is accepting not rejecting.

Love is: positive not negative. And we know that in all things God works for the good of those who love him (Rom 8:28).

I can do everything through him who gives me strength (Phil 4:13).

These verses, and others, underline the fact that faith in the Lord Jesus Christ is a positive faith. He gives us a constructive love for the world of men and women, through his Holy Spirit. A love that sees beyond the sinful negatives to the positive, godly potential of any redeemed life.

A paraphrase of 1 Corinthians 13 helps us realize the demands that this love makes upon us.

Love is inexhaustibly patient.
Love anticipates a person's needs and meets them.
Love doesn't mind when someone else has the limelight, responsibilities, popularity or privileges.
Love is not anxious to impress.
Love does not blow its own trumpet.
Love is not aggressive, but courteous.
Love does not insist on its own way.
Love is not touchy, or easily rubbed up the wrong way.
Love keeps no list of faults and failings of others.

Love doesn't gloat over the mistakes of others, in order to
   put itself in a better light.
Instead it is glad when others are right.
Love throws a cloak of silence over what is displeasing in
   other people.
Love trusts that in everything God works for good.
Love looks forward to the future glory promised by God.
Love is not shaken even by the worst of storms.
Love is eternal.

If you think that's difficult, you're wrong. It's impossible! Unless God helps us.

My husband Doug served for a spell in the Royal
Navy. During a visit to the West Indies his ship needed
refuelling. The Royal Fleet Auxiliary oil tanker came
alongside and the two ships harmonized their rate of
knots. A line was fired from the tanker and taken on
board the flagship. That line was attached to a steel
hawser and to that the oil pipe. When the latter was in
place, oil flowed from the heart of one ship into the
other. With the tanks now filled, pipes and hawsers were
returned and the flagship sailed on in the power it had
been given. It moved on because of another's provision.

Have the responsibilities and demands of family life
and marriage depleted your reserves? Then attach yourself to God. Take into your life the fulness of his Spirit.
Discover that the fruit of the Spirit is love. God's love
through you to others. Sail on in the provision of
another. You can face all that the future holds because
he will empower you to do so.

11

FIT TO SHARE

An early start, but a very pleasant drive, brought me to the old English pub in Buckinghamshire. This was the venue that had been hired by a Lunch and Dinner Club for the express intention of sharing the good news about Jesus. With comfortable seats and the smell of coffee greeting them as they arrived, the ladies noticeably relaxed. In familiar surroundings they readily listened to my talk on 'Fit for Life'. Questions and discussion and more coffee followed the talk. Then, as we neared the conclusion of the event, an attractive young woman hesitantly broke in on the discussion. She related that she had come to faith in Jesus Christ five weeks previously. Her enthusiasm and excitement were obvious. But with a shattering sentence, she wound up her short story 'Jesus must be the world's best-kept secret!' Those words have remained with me ever since. While we keep our mouths shut about Jesus and the life he gives us we play straight into the devil's hands. Jesus said, 'Go into all the world and preach the good news to all creation' (Mk 16:15). Although those words were spoken to his disciples many years ago, they remain valid for disciples today. Those words are also emphasized in Matthew

28:19-20. They are the greatest uncancelled commission of the church. Harold St John said;

> The chief business of every Christian in the world today is to evangelize. No consideration of age or sex, poverty or rank, allows you to escape . . . the controlling thing that lies before you is that your business in the world is to preach the gospel to every creature.

Evangelism is the proclamation of the gospel either publicly or privately, for the purpose of bringing men and women to faith in Christ as Saviour and Lord. In the early days of my Christian life similar statements struck fear into me. I struggled to obey this challenge to 'go into all the world'. These words triggered off a stream of grand ideas in my mind. I imagined packed stadiums, smoke-filled coffee bars, and pioneer missionary work. I realized that if this was evangelism it was only the especially gifted few who could fulfil such marching orders.

The masses of ordinary, insignificant Christians like me would have to continue to struggle on as best we could in our local situations. Ephesians 4:11 makes it clear that evangelism is the special gift of some. But it is also the constant duty and responsibility of us all. Only a few men and women will be called upon to proclaim the gospel publicly to huge masses collected together in soccer stadiums or air-fields. But that fact does not exhaust the possibilities for evangelism. Many of us identify with Jonah. God said 'Go' and he went. . .in the opposite direction, clouds of dust flying up from his disobedient heels. But he wasn't the only one who had agonies of heart and mind over God's instructions. Moses debated with God. Jacob wrestled with God. Peter impulsively promised to follow Jesus even to death, then found he couldn't. In identifying with Jonah, we can appreciate what Becky Manley Pippert has to say in her book *Out of the Salt-Shaker* (IVP 1980):

> There was a part of me that secretly felt evangelism was something you shouldn't do to your dog, let alone a friend.

Evangelism isn't something we do out of ice-cold duty. It is a way of life. A natural and spontaneous overflowing of the life of Jesus from us to our neighbours, family and friends.

At school during my teen years, there was a loud, extrovert member of our class who was forever dreaming up special boyfriends. She kept us amused for hours with her fictitious accounts of dates with these non-existent handsome hunks. We continuously challenged her to introduce these boys to us! We wanted to see them in order to believe her! Similarly, in introducing Jesus to our friends, neighbours, and workmates, we must make him visible through our lives. We are to be their Living Bible.

When Philip heard the angel of the Lord's command, he left his 'Mission Samaria' and went to one man out in the desert as he had been directed (Acts 8:26-40). What made Philip fit to share the good news of Jesus with an Ethiopian eunuch? It was because he was prayerfully tuned in to God. His relationship with God was current and the Holy Spirit controlled him. Prayer was a way of life to him, so when God said 'go' he went, and when the Spirit said go, he ran!

Philip was undoubtedly familiar with the voice of God. His preaching in Samaria had been accompanied by 'miraculous signs' (Acts 8:6, 13). Evil spirits were cast out of many and paralytics and cripples were healed (v.7). With its fascinating insistence on understatement, the scripture goes on to state, 'there was great joy in that city' (v.8). That was some crusade. Then slap bang in the middle of that action, Philip gets his instructions to leave the crowds in the city and go out into the desert. Stranger still—he goes. Why? Because he knows this is God's command. How? He recognizes the voice of deity. He's familiar with it. He doesn't put it all down to tiredness of mind. Nor does he feel he must stop eating dates and drinking goat's milk before going to sleep at night! He knows the voice that speaks to him. He's heard it before.

We were on holiday in Devon and were spending a day on the beach at Teignmouth. Stephen and Duncan were playing happily with other children, within our sight, at the water's edge. Just after midday, we decided our lunch could wait no longer. I asked Doug to call the boys to come for their sandwiches! Doug yelled out their names. Their little heads jerked up at the sound of their names ringing across the beach. They located the direction of the voice and galloped towards us. Above the noise of all the voices around them, they recognized the voice of their father and responded to it. They knew that voice by experience. They had heard it before.

Philip acted in obedience to a well-known voice. He was no spiritual oddity, nor evangelical freak. The Holy Spirit may use Christian eccentrics but he never creates them. Are you familiar with the voice of God? Can you distinguish his voice above the voices of friends and fellowship? Are you in tune with God? Able to obey swiftly and confidently his directions? The end product was that a sovereign, guiding God led Philip, the obedient servant, to the man seeking help with his questions.

Evangelism takes place when the people who know Jesus tell the people who don't know Jesus about Jesus!

This is not something to be manoeuvred, with all the accompanying striving, tension, anxiety and guilt. We do not need to invent avenues for evangelism. We can start from the basis that we are people with answers and need to be guided by God to meet people with questions. Just as God brought Philip to the African's chariot, he can bring you across the path of those who need to hear what you have to say! Ask God to do that daily and be on the alert for your special chariot, not just any old chariot!

When we take prayer and God seriously, we must be ready for surprises. My biggest surprise came last year. I was leafing through my prayer diary, making adjustments and adding answers and listing requests. This is one of my favourite exercises as I list in my prayer diary the personal encouragements as well as the disappointments. Glancing down at the Friday list with its requests and answers, I noticed the names of our previous neighbours. They had recently moved away. As I altered their address I also inserted the names of the young couple and their family, who had taken their place in the house next door. At about the same time a new milkman had also arrived. Down he went on the same page for prayer. From that day God increased my concern for those three people, but strangely my opportunities for speaking to them seemed to decrease. I saw very little of all three even though I prayed for them and sought to see them. One day I was called into their kitchen to be told that both husband and wife had become Christians and that the husband had led the milkman to the Lord! I am learning slowly that the question is not, who can I reach for God, but who can God reach through me? He is not always going to use me directly, but through my prayers, my life, my words, controlled by his Holy Spirit, God will work in his time.

The strength and encouragement that thousands have gained through the Mission England prayer triplets has been seen in changed lives and renewed Christians. There is nothing magic about the number three. The power lies in individuals uniting a whole country in prayer. A network of small prayer groups saturated our little island. As a consequence, hundreds of cared for and prayed for people came to know Jesus as their living Lord and Saviour, long before the visits of Billy Graham and Luis Palau. This work continued throughout their stay. If revival is to continue we must individually as well as collectively get down on our knees for our nation. Let's learn to pray for whole towns, villages and communities, as well as individuals. We must dare to sincerely ask God to give us a burden for our land and then we will know what it is to pray!

Although evangelism starts with prayer it must not stop there. Prayer and evangelism are hand-holding partners. Each natural opportunity to share Jesus should be initiated by and saturated in prayer.

As our love and burden increases for those we are praying for God will show us the importance of building relationships. Jesus was totally taken up with people. He loved them, spent time with them, and he had compassion upon them. Wherever he went they were naturally attracted to him. The common people, the working classes, heard his teaching gladly. If this Jesus lives in us, are people naturally attracted to us? Are we making Jesus 'visible, desirable, and intelligible' as Len Jones once put it so aptly. If not, why not? Too often our Christian lives are so boring we drive people away! In order to get close to people we need to be really interested in them. That means wanting to spend time with them and listening to them. It sometimes takes a very long time to earn the right to share with them. Many of us need to ask God to reveal again to us the tremendous news that Jesus is to the world!

After what seems to be a long wait through the summer months, thousands of teenagers eventually receive their exam results. Others wait patiently and hopefully for letters telling them that they have been employed, accepted on a course of special study, or for an apprenticeship. When the news is good the message is received loud and clear with the cheers, leaps of joy, hugs, sighs of relief, or a quiet look of contentment. To show others the slips of paper with the results is hardly necessary. The joy is obvious. Those who receive bad news communicate their disappointment and frustration in tears, silence and anger. We can all remember the sick feeling in the pit of the stomach as a result of failure, and the exhilaration of success.

If all that the Bible says is true, Jesus is the best news we can ever receive and pass on to others. With Christ's life in us, we are not failures. We're not beaten. Death isn't the end, we qualify for Eternal Life! A life that is full and exciting, not dependent on exam results and promotion. It relies on the tremendous sacrificial love that God has for us. Some of us have become so familiar with the fact of future eternal life that we have completely missed out on the present experience and excitement of it. The 'here and now' experience makes our sharing so much easier. Let us relax in the company of friends and share naturally our up-to-date experience of Jesus. Too many of us, because of anxiety, aggression and embarrassment, communicate bad news, even though our words may contain all the correct verses, facts and clichés.

The prayer triplet I belong to has strengthened all three of us considerably. We come from different churches, homes and neighbourhoods. We work together, pray together, and occasionally travel together. One long journey to the West Country saw us pull in for coffee at a wayside café. We talked through the day of seminars we were to be involved in. One took the role of a newcomer who hadn't a clue what she was coming to, whilst the others explained to her, without hassle, what it was all about. By accident and in fun, we discovered what 'learning situation' role play can be. In an easy, tension-free atmosphere we can listen to what we must sound like to a stranger and try to appreciate how a person who doesn't yet know Jesus must feel. If we are not used to talking about the Lord amongst Christians, how can we possibly expect to share him naturally with those who don't know him?

As we relate to others we are going to discover their special interests and hobbies. Those particular subjects which literally set personalities alight with enthusiasm. It was from a cross-section of the interests of our friends that a group of us produced our first programme for a monthly Friends and Neighbours evening. The subjects we covered ranged from a sportswear fashion show to a visit from an after care consultant, who spoke on the prevention, cure and after care relating to a mastectomy operation. Where there was a need, we included it in the programme. Hidden skills and talents were discovered amongst our friends and we encouraged them to share such skills as working in leather, computers, cookery and woodwork. To start with we met in my lounge, but as the group grew in numbers, we had to move to our chapel lounge. The togetherness we experienced in discovering and understanding each other's interests has naturally included sharing with the group more about Jesus. There has been cultivated amongst us a trust that does not simply look into the hobbies, work and interests of our friends, but also looks into the Bible to see what God has to say.

We quickly discovered that some needs were too big to be included in a monthly meeting alone. The needs of Mums with young toddlers and babies have been answered in a weekly playgroup and a monthly discussion time. Subjects including post natal depression, disciplining of our children, marriage and the family have been studied from a biblical point of view. A last minute fun evening included a Keep Fit session which broke more ice in relationships and led to a weekly keep fit class which has strengthened the link between our church and the neighbourhood. It is important in any relationship to feel secure, and it is heartening to see everyone joining in when and where they are able.

Are you moving into a new area? Think about the impact Jesus had on towns, villages, and streets as he moved in and around them. As you move into that house, flat or cottage, Jesus who lives in you also moves in. Some friends of ours, a young married couple, made a real impact on the cul-de-sac they moved into. They established contact by inviting neighbours in for coffee or supper. Having created a network of relationships, they introduced the various couples to each other. For some this was first introduction even though they had lived alongside each other for years. From this beginning came informal Bible Studies together. Doug and I met some of these couples at a special dinner. The comment of one man impressed us deeply. Speaking about our friends and especially of the wife he said, 'Until she came to live amongst us, we lived separate lives in the cul-de-sac, we knew no one. She introduced us to each other and now we are like a family.' He went on telling us about the impact of one lady on all their lives. In effect he was saying 'she became Jesus to us all'.

Are you going away to study at college or university?

Does your job involve you in travelling? Along with the natural apprehension and anxiety, remember you're taking Jesus with you. Christ lives in you and therefore every person who comes into contact with you—whether sitting in the lecture theatre, shopping in the supermarket, riding on the bus or sharing your table in the café—has a chance to meet Christ in you. Let him flow naturally and spontaneously out from you to them.

From Africa to Australia, England to Ethiopia, all countries, classes, cultures and castes set aside times for eating, drinking and relaxing. Jesus as well as the early church recognized these as vital times for evangelism. So should we. Most of us like to share a meal with friends and it's often easier to meet new friends in such an atmosphere. Our methods need to be flexible, catering for the varying needs of different areas. The kind of meals will also vary to suit different likes and dislikes. During a mission in East London, my husband ran a special ethnic food evening. The foods of all the different national groups were represented and sampled by all attending. Filipino and Japanese, Chinese and Indian, Cockney delicacies of jellied eels and cockles, all were there. An opportunity was made during the evening to speak about Jesus to all who came. Through the eating, links were strengthened between neighbours. In houses, halls, hotels, restaurants, cafés and ballrooms—the possibilities for this type of outreach are limitless. In twos or threes, hundreds or thousands, rich and poor, city dwellers and countrymen and women, all can be contacted this way. Scattered through the gospels we find Jesus using such relaxed times to share God's message with those around him. Matthew, eager to introduce his new-found friend to his fellow tax gatherers, threw a banquet (Lk 5:27-31). Jesus accepted invitations to spend time in other people's homes where they are at ease and feel less threatened. A leading Pharisee in Luke 14 and Zacchaeus in Luke 19, amongst many others, had time to ask questions of and talk to Jesus. Jesus spent time with individuals regardless of their background or their reputation. The comment about Jesus that 'This man welcomes sinners, and eats with them' (Lk 15:2) was intended to be a derogatory one, but it was in fact a compliment! By sitting at the table with the outcasts, Jesus demonstrated his love and concern for them. As a result, they listened to what he had to say and followed him.

If the fast-food burger take-away shops can welcome all, so can we. Never forget, we've got something far more satisfying and lasting to offer, in the good news about Jesus.

12

FIT FOR THE FUTURE

Do not cling to events of the past or dwell on what happened long ago. *Watch for the new thing* I am going to do. It is happening already—you can see it now! I will make a road through the wilderness and give you streams of water there (Is 43:18-19 GNB).

I write this final chapter exactly a year to the week that a family was plunged into a wilderness of bereavement, sadness and pain. Twelve months of memories, grief, emptiness and loss have passed since I wrote down the facts concerning the long nights I spent with Joy. She was a brave lady who clung to the words:

For this reason we never become discouraged. Even though our physical being is gradually decaying, yet our spiritual being is renewed day after day (2 Cor 4:16 GNB).

A verse that was full of hope concerning the new spiritual life she had so recently experienced. Words which, in this age that emphasizes physical fitness, will jog us into serious thought about the life that doesn't decay or decline with the years. This is a life that grows stronger and deeper as it is fed by the spiritual nourishment found in the words of the Bible, strengthened by the regular exercise of sharing the good news, and developed through the exercise of time spent in prayer.

Isaiah reminds us that God is a God of the new. He does not deal in the secondhand, nor does he patch things up or make do. He operates in new things. When he created the universe, he created it new. Jeremiah encourages us with the fact that God's mercies are 'new every morning' (Lam 3:23). The people of Israel were promised a 'new heart and a new spirit' by the Lord (Ezek 36:26). The salvation of God made possible through the death of Jesus involved the shedding of his blood, which Jesus said was 'the blood of a new covenant' (Mt 26:28). Forgiveness involves men in the experience of a 'new birth' as Nicodemus learned late one night in a face-to-face counselling session with Jesus (Jn 3). As a consequence 'if anyone is in Christ, he is a new creation; the old has gone, the new has come' (2 Cor 5:17). Now as sons and daughters of God no longer separated from him by our sin, we have 'confidence to enter the Most Holy Place by the blood of Jesus, by a new and living way opened for us' (Heb 10:19-20). As we contemplate the future, we are able to consider the 'new heaven' and the 'new earth', to look forward to singing 'a new song' with the yet unknown and unseen millions in the faith family. He truly is 'making everything new' (Rev 21:5).

For Joy it commenced with her personal experience of new life. Ten months later her husband discovered the way through the wilderness to faith in Christ. Around the same time Andy, Joy's youngest son, saw his fiancée reach out to receive the life of God. Through that one life that was taken to glory and released from bodily pain and trauma, other lives continue to be touched.

In our moments of deep distress and anguish of spirit,

we cry out 'Why, God?' It is almost an impossible question to answer. But we pick up clues as we look back and see how the purposes of God have unfolded in our life.

Have you ever climbed in the Lakeland Fells or the mountains of Scotland? Maybe you've struggled and gasped your way to the top. At times it was sheer agony as you pushed one foot in front of the other. In parts you were almost climbing blind as you couldn't see beyond the next fifty feet up. Nevertheless you went steadily and painfully forward. At the summit, or near it, you paused to look down the way you'd travelled. You saw it clearly with all its twists, turns and bends. It was much easier to discern in retrospect. That's so like life. Guidance is something we look back on and then we understand more fully. We see the wisdom of God in all. As his perfect plan unfolds behind us! So we can trust him for the way ahead. Life's road is rough and the journey is rugged at times. It can also be very unfair and unjust. But we cannot afford the luxury of moaning and complaining about it. God the righteous Judge will set it all right in due course. We have to go on with the business of living, knowing that we are living within his sovereign grace and goodness and that he is working out all things for his glory in our spiritual development. So we must keep watching 'for the new thing I am going to do. It is happening already' (Is 43:18 GNB).

But there are obvious conditions we have to fulfil in order to experience these new things. 'Do not cling to events of the past or dwell on what happened long ago.' We have to forget past successes and failures. A new event demands total concentration and fresh preparation. It will bring new glories and achievements, praise and perhaps new record times. We have to prepare ourselves spiritually just as an athlete prepares himself physically and warms up before the start of a big race.

I recall the day I saw the beautiful Red Admiral butterfly struggle from the dull brown casing that had been its home and protection during its silent metamorphism. Eventually the bright scarlet creature was entirely free from its old life. Free to fly up into the blue sky. To look up into the sun. To gain a new perspective of earth. No longer did it have a cabbage high view of earth. Now it soared upwards and saw things as they truly were in relation to everything else. Flying not crawling, out of darkness into light. From prison to liberty. Yet some time passed before that tiny creature had dried its wings and was ready to fly. Long enough for me to contrast the stirring beauty of that quivering insect with the empty, dead, drab case lying useless at its side. When it eventually took flight, it left that limiting, cramped casing behind. It would be ludicrous to imagine that butterfly clinging to its empty cocoon. That would limit its progress, or even render it impossible. It would drag it down causing pain and discomfort. Sadly many who have received eternal life in and through the Lord Jesus Christ are still clinging onto the debris of past failure and hurt. Others carry bitter wounds, deep resentments, unhealed memories, feelings of rejection and an unforgiving spirit. We try in vain to lift ourselves free from such darkness and pain. As a result, the promise of a full, free and victorious spiritual life has a hollow ring in our ears. There is no short cut to holiness and victory. We have been created with the capacity for a full spiritual life and that capacity will only be realized when we are filled by the Spirit.

Just as the butterfly has to leave its cocoon and experience the freedom of flight for the first time, so must we stop clinging to and wallowing in our past failures and triumphs. There are risks attached to liberty but these are to be preferred to the security of a death cell. The reality of our new life is seen when we let go of our comforting failures which can become our security and gain us attention and counsel.

Ships are built to sail the oceans. To face storms. To carry cargo and passengers to their destinations. They can't do so if they remain safe in the harbour, secured to the jetty by restraining hawsers. To be real ships they must 'let go for'ard and let go 'aft', slip the ropes or wires and sail out into the ocean. Christian living involves letting go of the jetty and launching out into the deep with God. It's a risky business but it is the only route to true spiritual fulfilment.

Although it's a short word, 'new' is an eye catching and exciting word. Advertising agencies have recognized its commercial power to capture the attention of the consumer. Packages, bottles, tins, plastic containers by the score all use these three simple letters. New improved biological powders, new booster bleach, new computer toys, new lawn rakers, new instant porridge, new cuppa soup! As a result, hands reach out to shelves and then dig deep into pockets and purses for the cash to purchase the goods.

In this exciting age, new records are being achieved, new inventions introduced to us, new planets reached and incredible new surgical techniques used. Television programmes and daily papers are headed with that famous word NEWS which was created from the four points of the compass, North, East, West and South. As we listen and read, we are informed about new tragedies, triumphs, disasters and achievements.

Having lived in London most of my life, I started my teacher training thinking that the North was North London or north of the river Thames! My ignorance was soon exposed by two fellow students from Yorkshire. They decided to educate me in the beauties of the Dales.

Four of us went on a very enjoyable Youth Hostelling holiday, exploring Wensleydale. One memorable morning, we had set out early, our packs were on our backs and a fine drizzle was driving into our faces. Everything was quiet and still. This serenity was splintered by a sharp yell, which came from across the fields. This was followed by the head and shoulders of an old farmer appearing over a rough stone wall. He beckoned excitedly to us. We peered in the direction in which he was pointing and there, freshly born, was a wet, wobbly lamb. That's a sight I hadn't seen very often on Clapham Common or around the Elephant and Castle! What amazed me was the expression of pleasure and excitement on that old farmer's face. As a farmer he must have seen hundreds, maybe thousands of lambs born. Yet this one was very evidently just as special to him as the first one. New birth! Freshly baked bread, the first snowdrop, the smell of new mown grass, the first breath of spring, all strike chords in the hearts of the romantic among us.

There is, however, a completely different side to this little word that strikes concern and fear into all of us. The unknown elements of life shake our confidence as we tackle new jobs, move to new homes, start new relationships, and face new experiences. We disguise the symptoms, and cover up the nervousness, but very little can stop the cold fingers of fear gripping our hearts as we try to cope with new situations. Each year commences with this powerful little word being thrown glibly in all directions. 'Happy New Year' we proclaim to all and sundry with careless ease. Where appropriate, we follow it up with the relevant greetings card for new jobs, exam successes, homes and anniversaries.

How is it possible to face the future and be fit and

ready for all the new experiences, both rough and smooth, that lie unknown just around the corner?

All would be plain sailing if we could order each new day like we order bread, milk or a meal. As a family we have a favourite restaurant down here in Bournemouth. We visit it on special occasions. The subdued lighting and comfortable furniture and decor are ideal for a relaxed evening. As the waiters and waitresses hover attentively, I love ordering my favourite food and then taking plenty of time to eat the well-prepared meal. The evening is always a success because we choose the right venue, food and company. Life would be so different if we could choose what happened to us and the people we met. We could eliminate everything unpleasant and successfully avoid everyone who rubbed us up the wrong way! The menu of life isn't so orderly. It comes with the unexpected as well as the planned. Each day is a new adventure, and no matter how well organized we are, the day is never completely under our control. I can't order each new day for me but I can order a new 'me' for each new day. 2 Corinthians 5 verses 17 and 18 lays it out clearly for us:

> Therefore, if anyone is in Christ, he is a new creation; the old is gone, the new has come! All this is from God.

Traumatic is the word that best describes my first experience of flying. I was alone and travelling to Jersey. I appeared to be relaxed and excited about the trip, to my family and friends. But the truth is that I was hiding a blind panic.

I was used to being in control of my journeys. My legs, a battered bike and the occasional bus and train had carried me safely through the first twenty years of my life. Now as I gaped at this mass of metal standing on the runway, my lack of experience and understanding of aerodynamics nearly overcame me.

Along with my fellow passengers, I boarded the aircraft and found a seat. I strapped myself in very firmly and then I glanced around at my fellow passengers. They all seemed calm and relaxed which didn't help me. I was churning up inside. Looking back I realize that the discomfort was due in part to the fact that I was not in control of the situation. Stepping into that plane involved giving myself over to its protection and to the skill of our unseen pilot. I had never met him and was never to see him during the whole of that flight. Ignorance and mistrust were at the root of my agitation and unease. After take-off, I began to experience what flying was all about. My apprehension faded and the incredible fact that I was flying at 20,000 feet and moving at 300 m.p.h. dawned upon me. More so, I was doing all that safely inside a piece of mechanized metal tubing!

In Christ there is complete and utter safety. 'I give them eternal life, and they shall never perish; no-one can snatch them out of my hand,' said Jesus in John 10 verse 28. Joined to him we have his all-round fitness to enable us to cope with all the unwanted and unexpected incidents of life. Gradually, he is changing all the old things and replacing them with his new things. To face the future confidently as Christians involves us in the daily exercise of leaving behind us the past. Too easily and rapidly today can become yesterday. But if faith is to be up to date we must be watching for tomorrow because God commands us:

Watch for the new thing I am going to do! (Is 43:19 GNB).

What he is going to do, first of all, is give us a new purpose! To a world that has lost its sense of purpose, that constantly poses the questions 'who am I?', 'where did I come from?', 'what is my destiny?', Jesus says 'I have come that they may have life, and have it to the full' (Jn 10:10). With him in our lives we can tackle the nitty gritty of daily living. I don't exactly jump for joy at the prospect of scrubbing a kitchen floor, nevertheless, however mundane the task, we have a God who is intimately interested in anything that concerns us. From housework to business management, teaching to engineering, banking to the dole queue, wherever we find ourselves, God accompanies us and gives to us a sense of his unique purpose in it all. With his help we can be better neighbours, friends, teachers, colleagues, parents, teenagers and students. God makes the insignificant and ordinary meaningful.

Secondly, he gives us a new prayer. No longer do we need to mechanically recite prayers. I always carry my RAC Associate Membership Card when I am driving. One evening I was returning from London and I arrived at the Winchester by-pass just as the light was fading. The rush hour was in full flow. This is definitely not the best time to break down, but it was exactly at that moment that my rear axle decided to fall apart. I knew my card included the RAC recovery service, so fishing it out of my bag, I went in search of a telephone. My friend and I crossed two fields to reach some houses and were directed by the occupants to the nearest phone. Five minutes' walking brought us to it and the queue outside. Patiently I waited my turn, only to find I had no change! Eventually the right coins were found and a friendly and most welcome voice started to deal with my problem.

'Could we have your membership number?' Fumbling with my card I took a deep breath.

'H18A B0726/6678270/N'

'I'm very sorry, your card is just out of date!'

My heart sank at that response. After consultation with my husband, who was at home and had the current membership card, our predicament was very efficiently resolved. As we returned over the fields to the car, I was impressed afresh with the tremendous gift prayer is.

> Call upon me in the day of trouble; I will deliver you, and you will honour me (Ps 50:15).

This is God's invitation to us. No phone calls, membership numbers, computers, checks or delays. No engaged signals. No out-of-date cards. Just immediate, undivided attention from God. In him we have our immediate recovery service on the journey of life.

Thirdly he gives us a new power. The power that alone can enable us to turn from the 'old' and expect the 'new'. By ourselves we will look longingly back to yesterday and wish it were tomorrow. We will continually dwell on the sadness or the glory of the past. Through the power of the Holy Spirit, let us follow Jesus' example and fix our eyes ahead and never look back from the task God has given us to do. Dr Donald Coggan has said,

> When the Holy Spirit comes on men and women there is New Life. There is often disorder too. Untidy edges. But give me this every time if otherwise I have to put up with cold orthodoxy.
>
> (Quoted in *Through the Year with David Watson*, Hodder & Stoughton 1922.)

Fourthly, he gives us a new prospect. The future for many appears bleak and frightening. Earthquakes, famine, violence, strikes, sexual immorality and the possibility of nuclear war, all fill our newspapers and TV screens. About forty wars are being fought right now in the world! How can we face such a future? A missionary taking up his first post in Africa was met at the conclusion of his long trip by plane and train. The final stage of the journey to his colleague's house was completed on the back of a mule in complete darkness.

'Leave it to the mule', he was instructed, 'the animal knows the way and is completely trustworthy. Don't try and guide it!' Within a quarter of an hour, the lights of the house were welcoming them. After a refreshing night's sleep the new missionary was taken on a conducted tour of the Mission Station. Everything was new and interesting. Then his friend brought him to the edge of a dangerous precipice. As they peered over the host pointed out a narrow track half way down, which was just wide enough for a mule to negotiate. A sheer drop continued beneath the mule track. The new missionary's face paled as he was told that the journey they had made the previous night had been along that track. 'Can you now see why I told you not to guide the mule? He was surefooted and had been that way before. You were safe with him!'

When our lives are in God's hands, they are in the safest place. God is in control of our life and destiny. He knows the way. He sees what lies ahead in the future for us and will prepare and equip us for it. But we need to seek his advice about it. The one thing that we can be certain that our future holds is God. He is out there ahead of us preparing the way. Psalm 23 verse 2 says, 'He leads me. . .' The eastern shepherd never drove his sheep before him. He was always out there in front discovering the pitfalls and traps before the sheep arrived. We have a spiritual shepherd and guide. A caring leader who will lead us through the most disastrous times. He will go ahead of us. Are you uncertain of your future? Searching for a job? Moving house? Awaiting exam results? Fighting disease or coping with disappointment? Take heart. The Psalmist reassures us:

He will instruct him in the way chosen for him (Ps 25:12).

If we fear God and ask him for guidance each step of the way our future is safe and secure.

Lastly, as we look for these new things that God is going to do, he gives us a new peace. A realistic peace, within all our turmoil. A peace that is best described by the following.

> The storm was raging, the sea beat against the rocks in huge dashing waves. The lightning was flashing, the thunder was roaring and the wind was blowing. But the little bird was sound asleep in the crevice of a rock. Its tiny head tucked under its wing. That is peace, to sleep in the storm. In Christ, we are relaxed and at peace in the midst of the confusion, bewilderments and perplexity of life. The storm rages but our hearts have found peace at last.

Each new experience, however exciting or formidable, can be made to count for God, who has secured our future, when we tackle them with a clear purpose, specific prayer, his ever ready power, and the peace that passes all understanding (Phil 4:7).

I surveyed the floating water skis with apprehension. The super-confident instructor hailed me from the boat, to enter the water. I had chosen a day for my first lesson when the sea was breaking heavily on the shore. Instead of fumbling for the first time on the beach into the cumbersome strips of wood, I had to swim out beyond the breakers and clip them into place as I floated! That's easier written than done! With my heart sinking, I battled with one unco-ordinated leg, my foot firmly clipped into its ski. Plus the fact that my bright yellow life jacket was tangled with the other ski, causing me to somersault several times.

As I surfaced from the last contortion, and thrashed helplessly in the water, the motor boat appeared alongside me. Quietly and firmly the instructor's words reached me. 'Bend your knees up to your chest and keep the skis raised and parallel.' Following this instruction, my elongated feet suddenly became more manageable. Grasping the first stage bar, which was secured to the boat, I held it above my head and braced myself for what was to come.

'Just remember, keep your knees bent, arms straight, and eyes fixed straight ahead!' The words hit home as the engine burst into life. The powerful boat picked up speed as I struggled to raise myself. Pushing with all my strength, I automatically straightened my legs, pulling on the bar. After several stops and starts, I managed to stay on top of the water. The time had come to follow the boat attached to the minute bar and rope. My tumbles and mistakes were painful, two water-ski-width bruises appearing on my legs. In desperation I called out to the returning boat, 'That hurt! What am I doing wrong?'

The reply was to be the key to my eventual enjoyment of this water sport. I had been struggling up too soon using my own strength, instead of relying on the power of the boat to pull me. As a result all instruction had literally gone to the wind. Arms were bent, legs straightened, head dropped, and sinking I lost contact with the boat!

Because of sin life hurts! God provides the power, through the spiritual life he gives us, to overcome sin and the accompanying pain and discomfort. As we look to the future, both individually and collectively, let's make sure we have accepted God's gift of new spiritual life, and are growing fit and strong, relying on his power and following his clear instructions to see us through.

FIT FOR A KING

A body now prepared by God and ready for war,
The prompting of the Spirit is our word of command.
We rise, a mighty army, at the bidding of the Lord;
The devils see and fear, for their time is at hand.
And children of the Lord hear our commission,
That we should love and serve our God as one.
The Spirit won't be hindered by division,
In the perfect work that Jesus has begun.

Today's Christian Woman

by Ann Warren

Women are people too!

Married or single, professional or at home, today's Christian woman faces an identity crisis.

Ann Warren writes to encourage women everywhere to take a positive look at their roles in society and the church. Avoiding the treacherous extremes of women's lib on the one hand and male domination on the other, she points the way to a creative and fulfilling life, free from the pressures that come from ignoring the Bible's view of man and woman.

Ideal for discussion groups and personal reading, this book affirms the glory that God has given woman in His created order.

Ann Warren is a pastoral counsellor, freelance writer and editor, and a regular contributor on the TVS television programme *Company*. She is married with three children.

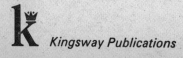

Kingsway Publications